Powerful Stories of People Living with
Depression, Anxiety, Addiction, Sexual Abuse
& Other Traumas

Made
to
Overcome

MENTAL HEALTH EDITION

Chou Hallegra & Friends

Made to Overcome - Mental Health Edition: Powerful Stories Of People Rising Above Depression, Anxiety, Addiction, Sexual Abuse & Other Traumas

Copyright © 2019

ISBN: 9798614860912
Published by Grace & Hope Consulting, LLC
www.graceandhopeconsulting.com

Project Leader: Chou Hallegra
Editor in Chief: Catherine Hughes
Graphic Designer: Shawnee Penkacik

Dedication

We dedicate this book to everyone facing mental health challenges.

Preface

Sixteen (16) men and women from different walks of life united to create this collaboration. They openly share how they are rising above depression, anxiety, addiction, sexual abuse, and other traumas.

Through their powerful stories, they want their readers to know:

There is hope. You are not alone; we are all in this together. Help is available. You can thrive in spite of what you've been through in your past.

When we don't talk about what troubles us, we increase stigma. When we don't talk about mental health, we reinforce the message that "we can't talk about it" - and that couldn't be further from the truth!

When we don't talk about mental illness, we increase the shame that people feel - shame caused by stigma. When people feel ashamed of their challenges, they don't seek help. When people don't seek help, bad things happen to them and to the people who love and support them.

It's time to break the stigma, one story at a time!
In our homes, let's talk about it.
In our schools, let's talk about it.
In our civic clubs, let's talk about it.
In our congregations, let's talk about it.
In every community, let's talk about it.

Table of Contents

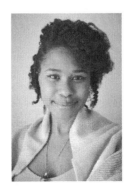

Karima Leslie

A Certified Spiritual Life and Business Coach, Karima Leslie provides one-on-one online and in-person coaching sessions for women all around the world.

She assists those seeking clarity in their life direction, guidance in improving their emotional & spiritual health, and action plans for those struggling to set & stick to daily goals. Karima's work has also been published in the anthology: *Driven: A Guidebook for Women by Women; To Inspire and Empower* and writes on topics involving self-doubt, overcoming trials, accountability, goal setting, making time work for you, self-acceptance, and creating a life you'll love.

Search for *Arise and Thrive Co.* on social media to

find her writing, free resources, and information about her services, or contact her directly at karima.author@ariseandthriveco.com.

Hope and Where to Find It: The Depression Antidote

By Karima Leslie

"...but we glory in tribulations also: knowing that tribulation worketh patience; and patience, experience; and experience, hope"

– Romans 5:3-4 KJV

What makes depression and anxiety so imprisoning is how it sucks you dry.

All your motivation, gone. Your will, gone. Your joy, gone.

Everyone tells you "it will get better." And they're right. But what people fail to mention is that things are not going to magically get better on their own.

It doesn't get better until *you* are the one to make things better for yourself.

Advice from those around you can often feel tone-deaf. The root of the problem seems to be consistently ignored. You didn't just bump into depression one day like an old classmate at the supermarket. Vitamin C and exercise won't bring back your loved one who passed away or give you a sense of direction when the kids have moved out of the house or fix the job you hate but pays the bills. So, you dismiss the advice, feeling even more hurt and misunderstood. And then you feel guilty for ignoring their suggestions. You know there may be some truth in their words but even if the advice they give is helpful, you still can't seem to pull out the necessary strength to act on it.

Everything seems more difficult with each passing day and your self-esteem slowly fades until you end up doubting your ability to do anything. Looming despair clings to your limbs like a ball and chain and you begin to put up emotional walls so that people don't see you like this. Brick by brick you build the cell that you'll eventually suffocate in.

There's a better way.

Your ability to focus is rare and fleeting so don't spend it pushing through a day of disordered activities that you hate, or around toxic people that just deplete you further, or on things that no longer bring you joy and are just a means of escape.

Your focus is precious, and you owe it to yourself to dedicate it to healing.

Healing may look different for you than it does for

others and that's ok because (and maybe you don't believe this yet, but) you deserve a life you can love. You deserve a life free from constant anxiety, stress, and sadness. You deserve a life where you love yourself and the environment around you.

It took going on my own journey through depression to truly believe that there was light at the end of the tunnel. It may be difficult, but it is so very worth it.

How It Started

One day, I woke up in a daze with a pounding headache. Early in the morning on my way to work, I felt like someone had stuck my brain inside a dryer as I went through my day feeling more and more nauseous, agitated, and faint.

I felt like that for two weeks until I finally went to the doctor and was eventually diagnosed with anemia - a blood condition ranging from mild to severe, easy fix to permanent. Six months and multiple different medications later left me feeling worse than I ever had before. The constant exhaustion and pain led me to believe that this was all I would ever feel. As I became oxygen deprived due to the anemia, tasks that I once completed on autopilot now took hours to perform and left me feeling like all my brain cells had abandoned ship. More accurately, my brain cells, along with all my other organs, were being held hostage and refused the air they needed to function.

With no mental or physical energy, depression slid inside me without me ever noticing its silent intrusion. Slowly filling my being with its poison, it whispered new thoughts that scared me:

"No one will ever figure out what's wrong."

"It's hopeless."

"If the rest of my life is going to be spent in pain, then I don't want to be here for it."

Depression invited a friend in one day, or maybe she was always there to begin with, but now felt emboldened. Her name was anxiety, and she burrowed under my skin. Each day, she burned a little hotter.

"It's been too long since I've worked. But every time I work it kills me. My savings are draining away. What happens when it's all gone? How will I pay my bills? How long will it take the landlord to kick me out? Who will take care of me if I keep getting worse? I must be painfully boring to talk to. Does my boyfriend hate me now? Probably, he's lost interest in me. I miss my friends. Conversations are awkward. I'm just a downer. I never leave the house. I have nothing to talk about anymore. I'll answer the phone when I feel better."

Everything had gotten too hard. I would go through times of not wanting to speak to anyone and desperately needing someone to talk to. "I'm tired" didn't really get the point across. Neither did "I'm in pain" or "I'm sad" but everything felt too muddled and too new for me to explain properly. I convinced myself that further elaboration would be too much information that no one wanted and replies of "No" to the question "Are you ok?" seemed to shut down most conversations.

More months of feeling hopeless and out of control went by without me realizing that while my illness was still an everyday struggle, anemia was no longer the thing threatening me the most. At a certain point, I had mentally given up. "*Nothing will ever change*," I thought. So, I stopped trying. I stopped looking for new treatments, stopped trying to be happy. I stopped my obsessive search for control and faded from the woman full of life to mere existence.

It wasn't until I got my hope back that I saw any point in trying again. **Hope was the turning point that brought me back from barely existing, to passionate about life again**. I was lucky to find a glimpse of hope, knowing many people around me who hadn't gotten theirs back in years. But it didn't come easily, even when it felt like I was stumbling upon it, each fragment of hope felt like finding a buried piece of treasure on a year-long scavenger hunt. So, I started to map it out.

The Thing About Hope

Hope is a slippery thing, but this is what we know:

Not just something reserved for the religious or the overly optimistic, hope is a necessary element in a healthy mindset. It's the part left out far too often when we talk about motivation and drive. **Hope is what pushes us forward, allowing us to *want* to keep going**. It fights against the negative voices in our ears and hearts and tells us to pick ourselves back up and keep going.

Happiness is to sadness what hope is to fear, and fear is rooted deeply in depression. There is fear that things will never change, fear that you're not good enough, fear that things will keep getting worse, fear that you're powerless over what happens to you, and fear that you'll be forever stuck in a pit of despair with no way out.

But **hope helps us envision what we would desire and grants us the confidence to make it happen.** It tells us that change is not only possible but probable. Hope is the key to being able to handle the problems life throws at you and still remain confident and resilient. **When faced with obstacles, hope clears a path to make it through, providing the motivation necessary for healing, building, and maintaining a**

satisfying life.

Hope is the glue that we need to piece our hearts back together no matter how badly we've been broken or how deeply we've been defeated. That's why, when we lose that hope - our glue - we feel like there's no point in collecting the pieces without anything to make them stick.

How We Lose It

We can lose our hope for different reasons:

An Unexpected Event

Something happened or was done to you that you didn't see coming - abuse, natural disaster, illness, discrimination, death of a loved one, unfair treatment, etc. In events such as these - once and / or ongoing - we begin to feel like we no longer have control over our situation or what happens to us. The perceived loss of control can lead us to feel like bad things will happen to us by merely existing and that it's pointless to try for things when we feel like a spectator in our own lives.

A Loss of Identity

You suffer an injury and can no longer pursue your passion, or your kids move out of the house and all of a sudden, your purpose seems gone. The core of who you are is altered. You had worked for years putting huge amounts of time, energy, and effort into one thing and then you lose it. It was what you loved and what you were good at and the void it leaves is soul-crushing. Now that thing is gone, and what do you do with yourself? Not only that, but why bother starting all over again with something new that may bring you less happiness and pride? You feel lost, like you're floating from random task to random task with no significance to it all. With more and more things seeming meaningless, you lose your joy and stop most of your previous activities.

Overwhelm & Burnout

You work yourself to the point of exhaustion, wearing busy as a badge. But now all your to-dos and work and appointments and meetings seem never-ending and stack up to the point where you feel unable to handle anything anymore and things start to unravel. It feels like life has run you over and all your responsibilities weighed so heavily upon you that eventually, you broke down, unable to cope, and everything came to a roaring stop with no foreseeable way - or desire - to start back up again.

For me, it was a combination of all three. Almost a year before I was diagnosed with anemia, I suffered from **burnout** at my job. Working for a large corporate agency, I was expected to be available 24/7 should any issue arise. There were always issues to deal with, always fires to put out and I would receive emails and text messages stating "911" from upper management as if a fellow coworker calling in sick was a life or death emergency. Eventually, my contract ended, and, happy to leave, I took up a part-time position and started my own business at the same time. When I wasn't working for someone else, I was working for me, and hobbies and free time became non-existent. I began to work myself into the ground which undoubtedly was the catalyst to my declining health.

And then my illness came, **an unexpected event** that I didn't see coming because I wasn't paying attention. I wasn't in tune with my body's needs, ignoring how burnt out I was and trying to push through it without addressing it. I was continuing to work 12-14 hour shifts even though I desperately needed rest - until my body finally broke down in its final cry of "*enough!*"

When that happened, and I physically couldn't work anymore, a large part of my **identity was fractured**. I had always prided myself on the fact that I not only "got stuff done" but that I was an overachiever, managing to do everything all at once and juggle it perfectly. I had started overworking as far back as university.

In school full-time, I still held multiple part-time jobs and would end up skipping classes just to work and then pulling all-nighters to ensure my grades wouldn't slip. By doing this, my $30,000+ student loan debt was paid off a few months after graduation. I finished university with honors and came out with both a four-year Bachelor of Commerce degree with a major in marketing and a two-year specialty diploma in Asia Pacific Management in an accelerated program at the age of twenty-two. At 23, I had gotten a diploma in photography and graphic design, travelled abroad for a bit, taught English and was a tourism intern in China which I counted as vacation.

At 24, I was being asked by companies to travel around Canada for client work and had six years of working experience in marketing. I also became certified in Spiritual Life Coaching and started my own company the same year, as a Spiritual Life and Business Coach.

I was complimented a lot - over and over - on how great my work ethic was, and how good I was doing, and how I had an amazing ability to keep it all together. That hustle mentality became the majority of who I was. "*Of course, I can do it all because that's just who I am.*" I was Karima, and that's just the kind of stuff Karima did.

Then the anemia came, and gone was my identity.

I was frustrated that my body was failing me and felt trapped in my own house as all my hopes and dreams fell by the wayside. There was so much that I wanted to do, and I couldn't do any of it. I no longer felt like the girl who could do it all but instead, the woman whose body had given up.

My **overwhelm** grew as no medication or treatments seemed to have any effect and only made me worse.

"What's the point of continuing to try?" This hope draining cocktail (loss of identity, unexpected events, and overwhelm and burnout) had beaten me. When that happened, and everything felt too heavy for me to carry, my saving grace was being honest about how I was feeling and gaining a new perspective.

Point One: Breaking Tunnel Vision

I first talked about it with my boyfriend, then my friends, and eventually my family. I spoke about how hopeless I felt, that I would never get better, and that I hated living like this. I argued my tired opinion that there was no point trying anymore.

"You're not going to be like this forever."

"This is just a tough period."

"You've gotten through tough situations before."

"It's not always going to feel this tough."

They pointed out that I had the ability to adapt, each in their own way - and this was a liberating thought. They reminded me that there were still so many things we hadn't tried and that I would be

13

healthy again, and **even if things never went back to the way they were, I would still be ok.** I would start to understand my new parameters and things would slowly feel less hard and I would adapt to my new circumstances. **So crucial were these thoughts; they revived my faith** - faith that things could be good again. They gave me faith to try.

I had gotten so focused on my current pain that I equated continuing to try with prolonging how awful I felt in those painful moments. In my mind, there were only the two extreme outcomes: either my illness went away immediately with everything going back to normal (which seemed highly unlikely), or my body and mind would continue to deteriorate, and life would remain impossible. I could see no other possibilities.

But with this new thought: *I could adapt.* **I was broken out of my tunnel vision**.

Then there was the second problem - I doubted my ability. I knew that in the past I had overcome trials but, in the past, I also had energy. I no longer felt like that girl anymore and I didn't know if this "new me" had what it took. This brought me to the next point in my journey.

Point Two: Acceptance, Patience, and Love

Once the idea had been planted that I could adapt, I started doing the activities I used to enjoy before I was ill. I tried going back to work, cooking, running errands, exercising, and writing. Most of it went miserably. I didn't have the physical and emotional capabilities I once had and tasks that I could usually do with little effort now took hours and left me drained.

Again, I opened up about how I was feeling and had a valuable talk about the importance of being patient with myself. I was in a new season in life that had different rules than I was used to and new constraints that were not only physical but emotional and spiritual as well - and that was ok. If I only had a limited amount of energy, it meant my energy was precious and should be used wisely. If certain tasks were too hard, then I needed to learn to ask for help. If there was a limited amount of time in the day where I could function, then I would try not to push it past that amount of time.

I was reconnecting with my body and its needs, learning to be patient, and working within my new parameters. **I had to learn to love myself again and remember that my worth was not connected to the number of things I could get done in a day or how many achievements I could make in a year**. My frame of reference needed to change from thinking about all the things I was able to do in the past, to finding appreciation in what I was able to do now, in the present, given my constraints - even if that meant just going grocery shopping or cooking dinner.

Point Three: Learning From Experience

The more I got to know myself the easier things became. I learned how much time I usually had in a day to function and planned accordingly. I searched for things to lighten spirits on bad days and paid attention to my needs (physically, mentally, & spiritually) and learned how to fulfill them. I also learned what things fed my sadness or anxiety and how to diminish them, what would trigger my overwhelm and how to find calm, how much sleep my body needed, what foods made me feel worse, and who I could talk to about my depression & anxiety. These were things **I learned over a long stretch of time and through trial & error. But learning to be mindful, to pay attention to what I was feeding my soul, was an exercise that made me feel like I was moving forward, and this was incredibly important**.

Point Four: Momentum, Trust and Hope

"Tribulation worketh patience; and patience, experience; and experience, hope."

This is a passage I never truly understood until I had lost hope and went on a journey to find it again. Our trials and tribulations either break us or we learn to be patient in them, with ourselves and with situations beyond our control. Through our patience, we gain experience and we learn how to function in the midst of depression. But it was the last part of the passage that made me stop and ponder how that connected to hope. I continue to delve into this topic today and have become fascinated with hope.

As a Spiritual Life and Business Coach, I've learned from my own journey, my client's journeys, and my loved one's journeys - that hope follows when we start to take action and feel that our actions, experiences, and learnings will help us move forward in life. When you see that you're progressing and not deteriorating - making decisions and not just spectating - you're motivated to keep going. Because you're progressing, you can more easily trust that you won't be in this dark place forever. With that growth and momentum comes hope for a brighter future.

After this comes trust. For me, as someone who's heavily spiritual, trust came in the form of radical surrender to what I call God. It was trusting in something bigger than myself to the point that whatever happened around me or to me, I would be ok, and my world would be ok. It was trusting those negative situations and events could be used for good and I could come out stronger. I was learning how to work in God's timing, a plan that did not have me as the sole lead on stage but as a character given their time to shine, as well as their time in the shadows. I learned that all seasons of life, bright and dark, were needed to build that character and would be useful later on in their story. I learned how to be more patient and less self-centered, how to utilize my time and energy more efficiently, how to cope with anxiety, how to overcome self-doubt, and how to grow in self-love and spirituality. My story could help others who were going through similar things, feel less alone. And for that, I am grateful.

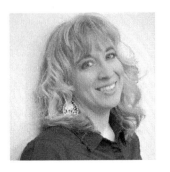

Catherine Hughes

Hailing from southeast of Pittsburgh, Pennsylvania in a small town recently dubbed as "the most boring town in Pennsylvania," Catherine Hughes is the daughter of two English professors. She is a passionate advocate, innovative storyteller, and community strategist.

For over 15 years, she has provided comprehensive support and passionate advocacy to individuals and self-advocates, their families, and surrounding natural supports throughout their communities. She considers herself a servant leader, one who cultivates, develops and maintains relationships with grace and grit in order to create, enhance, and promote services and programs that transform lives. On a personal level, her calling (not a career) allows her to give back some of what has so graciously been given to her family.

19

Catherine is currently participating in several writing collaborations (leading two as the editor), and also finishing up her first solo publication, *Imprisoned No More*. She manages a blog and social media platforms as *The Caffeinated Advocate.* She is also a sought-out trainer and speaker.

Living with her in that boring town but not so boring household are Mama Betty, Christian, and their pets Callie, Cookie, Candie, Hannah, Maddie and Raven the Cats, and the one and only Abby Dog.

Blooming Through Rocky Soil

By Catherine Hughes

"Keep your face to the sunshine, and you cannot see the shadows. That's what sunflowers do."

~ Helen Keller

Anyone who knows me quite well knows that I love coffee (I mean, I am The Caffeinated Advocate) and sunflowers. About six years ago, I attended a gala supporting a grassroots organization in the autism community. One of the entertainers of the evening was a relatively well-known psychic. I was pretty excited to get my reading and was uber-curious to hear his insight.

"Sunflowers. They are important to you, no?" he said.

"Yes, they are," I said incredulously, tears stinging my eyes.

Silk sunflowers sat in a modest glass vase on my desk in my office - the last item I grabbed from my grandparents' mantle before I closed the door of their home one final time. 113 10th Street was my safe haven as a child. During times of struggle throughout my childhood and even my pregnancy with my son, "Ma and Papa's" (my mother's parents) house was like an escape for me, not to mention the site of many holiday dinners and gatherings for our small family.

"You must not ever ignore signs of change coming or the opportunity to embrace something perhaps scary but new when you see them or hear of them. These are your Avatar, your Venus or Oshun. You ARE a sunflower," said the entertainer.

In the last few years supporting my own family and communities through my work, as well as pushing through my own recovery, I now know exactly what he meant by being a sunflower.

Five years ago when I was deeply struggling with my own mental health, I received sunflowers from my boss and his partner, with the quote from Helen Keller that I shared above on the enclosed card. After decades of tragedies and triumphs, this quote is one I carry with me in everything I do - and that card also sits on my desk with Ma and Papa's old silk sunflowers.

I'm the daughter of two English professors, one of which turned postal carrier (that would be my Daddy) shortly after I was born. It was not long after his father's sudden death (Dad was in his early twenties) that he was diagnosed as bipolar, back then more commonly known as manic depression. Throughout my childhood, he was institutionalized about every two years. Even as a young girl, I came to learn that when my father would go to the canvas on our wall and talk about when he painted it for a gallery, began fiercely writing poetry during all hours of the night, or using alcohol heavily and more frequently to self-soothe rather than take his medication, something was amiss and it was time for Dad to leave again for thirty-some days.

When I was ten, my father enrolled in a treatment program. I'll never forget the day he came home. I was in the hallway standing between two of my fifth-grade teachers, and they said "It's a BIG DAY for Cathy!" I couldn't stop talking about his homecoming. I thought ceasing alcohol consumption might prevent future episodes. Unfortunately, at that tender age, I didn't know just how lifelong and profound his diagnosis truly was.

Unable to deal with both the pressures from home and from those at school who made me feel like I just wasn't good enough, I turned to crash dieting at the age of twelve. I certainly felt smart enough, but I also felt like the four-eyed fat nerd, to be frank. I wasn't pretty enough despite the smashing wardrobe my parents spoiled me with in spite of our lack of financial wellness.

23

And goodness knows, I wasn't skinny enough. Not like "the other girls!" I lost over thirty pounds in a three-month period and I was headed towards the double digits on the scale. I began passing out frequently after exercising for hours on end and living on salad and popsicles. I ended up at the hospital multiple times - one time, I was taken out on a stretcher from the local mall. It was then that a doctor came into the cubicle where I was on yet another IV drop, and he said, "Enough is enough. You honestly have two choices - start eating and obtain a healthier weight, or you're going to end up in a program."

I was frightened to death about being taken from my family and knew that I had no choice but to stop my anorexic behaviors. I came to my senses and slowly began to accept myself for who I was. In the ninth grade, I gave a speech to my language class about my experience as a pre-teen with an eating disorder. I received a standing ovation and many teary-eyed thank you's from other girls. I also was given many apologies from those who thought they had ever made me feel less than.

My journey was far from over. Also, learning of other family members suffering from schizophrenia, obsessive-compulsive disorder, Alzheimer's and others who abused substances, living with a parent who had manic depression was still a battle, though he was becoming more stable for longer periods of time.

At the age of 15, my date sexually assaulted me on our way home from a semi-formal Valentine's Dance. It happened in the back of the vehicle belonging to the sister of the gentleman who later became my high school sweetheart. My perpetrator also physically assaulted me by choking me against a locker weeks later, after I threatened to go to both the principal and the authorities about what he did to me. After seeing marks on my neck, my boyfriend chased him down the hallway while I stood in tears, completely distraught and scared out of my mind. I learned that the principal was the best friend of my date's father. After sharing what I could remember about that night I was attacked by my date, while also showing him my neck, the only thing he said to me was this: "You must be a tough girl to get over." I still can't forget that moment to this day. I, the victim, was blamed.

I found myself pregnant in college at the end of my freshman year. Ditched and feeling remarkably alone, my boyfriend at the time (who happened to be the son of one of my mother's childhood best friends) had decided "he just didn't love me anymore" after I refused to have an abortion. This was a traumatic experience, so deeply disturbing that I just cannot describe it in words. Feelings of anxiety and depression were creeping in again more than ever. It was bad enough trying to tell my mother about this news, but my father? I was blessed that his reaction to my pregnancy was to leave the house, drive to the drugstore, and purchase a bib and a bottle that said: "I Love My Grandson." He came home, silently placed them in front of me on the coffee table and walked out of the room.

When my child was three, another trauma plagued our family. I was falsely accused of child abuse after a horrific misunderstanding in the community, and I was arrested and then jailed for days. The positive note - despite months of hearings and $20,000 lost - is that the situation resulted in my son receiving his diagnosis on the autism spectrum much faster than had I gone the typical route of getting a referral and waiting for an evaluation. This was one of the moments in my life that demonstrated to me that everything happens for a reason.

As I sought services and supports for my son, I was also working full-time and planning for a wedding. The marriage was short-lived - less than two years, in fact. It was six days before our second anniversary that I came home after a community event for families impacted by autism to find an empty basement (our bedroom at the time). I found an eight-page letter on my desk insisting on what a horrible person I was and why he needed to leave and now. My parents thought he was going bowling. Meanwhile, he packed his car with his belongings and told my son that "Mommy makes bad choices." It took months for me to repair that emotional damage.

While this storm continued to pour down, I was also a caretaker for many family members. My father became critically ill to the point of requiring a wheelchair and thus becoming deeply depressed. My grandparents, now in their 80's were very weak and needed help to maintain their home. They lived an hour away, so trying to commute and support them while also helping my mother to care for Dad and be the autism supermom managing my son's needs triggered my mental state. I sought a therapist and a psychiatrist who diagnosed me with panic disorder, anxiety, and depression (not to mention noting my history of disordered eating). I was seeing the therapist weekly but the roulette of medications took a toll on me. Symptoms became too much to bear and I tried to manage on my own.

By 2009, the year that my father was slipping away from us, my eating disorder resurfaced with a vengeance. I thought I was making healthy choices by "watching what I ate and working out," but the reality was, I needed something to control. I engaged in both anorexic and orthorexic behaviors, even throwing some bulimia into the mix. Anytime I felt like I "binged" (which was all in my head), I washed down laxatives and diuretics with water - just enough not to add more weight to my body.

27

I continued on this path for about three years before my new "a-ha" moment was presented. I had moments of passing out again like my adolescent days either from the two-hour workouts or laxative abuse. I remember one time passing out on the floor during a summer camp visit, dripping in sweat, and my colleague (who thankfully was also a dear friend) drove us back. Not long after, as my suffering became apparent to everyone around me, more and more colleagues approached my boss and asked for him to step in. He was (still is) not just a boss, but a confidante, mentor and truly family. I visited our office after a speaking engagement. He asked me to sit down, and he proceeded to give me the intervention I needed so very much.

"There are three phones here. Which one are you using to make an appointment for yourself?"

Weeks later, I went to my first appointment ever with the woman who proceeded to treat me for five years. I also threw up all over myself on the way home because I could not believe what came out of my mouth in those 55 minutes. "Why are you here?" was such a loaded question.

Throughout my past and current experiences with family, the communities I am blessed to serve, and myself, I know the importance of self-care and the importance of a support system. I know that I cannot reach my goals, or help others to achieve theirs if I am not at my best.

I've also learned that the diagnoses we have faced are out of our control and they are not anyone's fault, but the way we respond however, is. My mother, my son and I have to fight every day for our mental wellness and address them in different ways - from medication to music to meditation and so much more. We have learned that we are worthy of being well. We have learned that our labels don't define us, and that we define ourselves.

We were planted in rocky soil, but we still bloom. Throughout the shadows, we find the sunshine.

That's what sunflowers do.

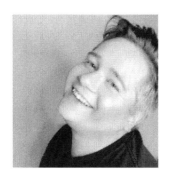

Thomas Newman Powell

Thomas Newman Powell of Loris, South Carolina is a graduate of Green Sea Floyds High School. He is the author of *Warrior: Songs of a Fighter*, a book consisting of poetry he wrote from ages 13 to 17 about his home life struggles, anxiety, and depression.

Thomas has released a solo music single titled *Post My Bail* that he composed alongside his mother. He also composed and performed a song with New York rapper Rxflo titled *Where Were You* which served as the lead single from the rapper's up and coming album *The Eulogy* which focused on the downside and loneliness of one-sided friendships and support during personal hardships.

In support of his music projects, Thomas has

appeared on local television and has received radio play in the Myrtle Beach area. He is a member and activist of the LGBTQ community, even appearing in one-off drag shows. He has been an active member of the state-recognized Waccamaw Indian People since being a child, in which his great Uncle serves as The Chief and other family members serve in council positions.

Thomas hopes to keep pursuing his dream of being a songwriter and musician as he continues to work on and release projects over time saying that "maybe by publicly expressing my struggles and truths, I can be the voice that the bullied kid in the corner may need to hear to know they are not alone. Never allow someone to dim your light. Look at all the things you can accomplish." Thomas can be reached at powellthomas2@gmail.com.

Finding My Rainbow

By Thomas Neuman Powell

"In the darkest time, I have always believed, the light will shine."

– Laila Gifty Akita

When I look back on old pictures or videos from my childhood, I can't seem to remember the happy times. My dad pushing me on the swing, blowing out the candles on my fourth birthday cake, or even the smiles and giggles I shared with my great-grandma who spent almost every day of my life with me before she died of leukemia. It's almost like I have blocked them out or they have been overruled by the trauma that came around the age of nine.

The very first memory that comes to mind is the night my mom left my dad. She shattered their marriage license on the floor and walked out of the house. Crying on the couch, holding my best friend "Spotty" a stuffed dog my great-grandma had given me before she passed, brought me comfort but it just wasn't enough.

During their divorce, my mom had gotten on the

wrong path and mixed in with the wrong crowd of drug addicts and bad influences. She got into an accident, broke her neck and almost lost her life. I remember that night my dad woke me up, and we rushed to the hospital. I put my hand on top of hers and asked, "Are you going to die?" She replied "No." I then asked her, "Do you promise?" She looked at me and said, "I promise." She had such determination in her eyes. At that time, she was the first and only successful recovery of that kind of neck injury at that particular hospital. That determination paid off because she kept her promise. She recovered, got clean and was remarried (to an officer).

While things got better with her, my dad became dependent on alcohol and took out his frustrations on the only person around: me. Some of the things he would say that bothered me the most were "you'll never be anything," "you're just like your mom," and "I hope you find a good man to take care of you because you will never make it on your own." Hearing those words coming from someone I loved and cared about hurt me so much. Mental abuse is unforgettable. To this day, those words are still hurdles I face daily.

He dated on and off and I had women or "parent figures" in and out of my life throughout my school years. It became hard for me to say the words "I love you," because once I started to love someone they would walk back out of my life. However, I'm thankful for every one of them. They each affected my life more than they know.

Every summer I would go to my grandma's, in the next town over, to "escape" from everything at home. At 16, one summer night turned into the night that permanently changed the way I saw myself. I met a guy on a social media platform. We talked for a while and even though he was 24, I didn't feel as if I were in danger. He asked if I would like to get together and play video games and watch movies. Being 16, bored at home on a Friday night, I agreed. Knowing that my grandma wouldn't agree with me leaving with a stranger, I told her I would have my friend from school pick me up and we would go out to a teen club in the area. She was fine with that but wanted me to bring her back Dubble Bubble chewing gum from a store on my way back. This was the first time I had lied to her or taken a risk.

At about 9 p.m., a beat-up station wagon pulled up in her driveway and I nervously got in the car. He seemed really nice and kept joking to get me to loosen up and stop being so shy on the way to his house. He seemed to be just like the personality he portrayed online. During the conversation, I told him I needed to pick up chewing gum from a store on the way home. He was fine with it and then explained that his father was out of town and he had the house to himself.

Once we got back to his home, he offered to make me a drink. At this time in my life, this was the first time I had tasted alcohol, but I accepted so I didn't look "uncool." We conversed for a while on the couch and then he said "My Xbox is in my room upstairs. If you want to go up, I'll meet you there in a minute." So I walked up the stairs. The closer I got to his bedroom door, the eerier I felt. It was like my mind was telling me to turn around. The other part of my brain was telling me I was just shy and needed to trust him and have fun. The stairs creaked with his footsteps behind me as I hit the top stair and I walked in.

He followed in right behind me and shut the bedroom door behind him. He paused, stared at me, and I saw him twist the lock. There was a strange look in his eyes, something I had not seen since he picked me up. At this point, the eerie feeling became so overwhelming I asked him if maybe we could go back downstairs and just watch TV and talk. He then got closer and closer, with every footstep my heart started to beat a little faster.

Once he got about a foot from me he said, "We aren't going back down." He took a step closer and he started to run his hand down my back. I explained that I was uncomfortable and would like to go back home. He then said four words that I'll never forget: "You're not going anywhere." I attempted to pull away from

35

him but he was well over 6 feet tall and me being only 5 foot 5 there was no match. In the tussle he said, "If you ever want to go back home, you will just do this!

Make it easy on yourself." He dragged me to his bed and raped me.

After the incident, he allowed me to shower. I remember looking in the mirror before I got in. I saw a teary-eyed, bruised-armed boy with messy hair. Once I got cleaned up, I got back in his car and he started to take me home. He said, "I'm going to stop and let you get the chewing gum." I looked over in such disgust. How did he even remember that I needed it? I sure didn't. That was the very last thing on my mind.

We pulled into the parking lot of a grocery store. He grabbed my arm and said, "If you say anything to anyone, I will slit your throat." Walking into the store he stayed right behind me. Inside I felt like running, crying, and screaming, but I was scared he would actually kill me. I grabbed the gum and proceeded to the checkout counter. He stood by the front door glaring at me with pure evil in his eyes.

The cashier rang up my item and asked how I was. The only word I could get out was simply, "Ok." She replied with "Hon, are you sure?" and looked over at him. I nodded. We got back in his vehicle and he drove me to my grandma's home. Before I got out of the car, he forced me to kiss him and said, "I'll see you again soon" followed by a wink.

As soon as I got in the door, I threw the gum on the counter, ran to the guest room and just cried until I couldn't anymore. He had my address! He could just come back anytime. What if he did? For nights, I stayed up worried that he would return and hurt me again.

Every time I looked in the mirror I felt disgusting and I hated everything about myself. I felt dirty - the kind of dirt that no shower could wash away. Internally, I was spread across so many emotional spectrums. Would the innocence and trust I had for people ever return? Or was I ruined for good?

Once school started again, I was called horrible names for being gay and because I was overweight. I only had a handful of friends and I felt embarrassed to talk about the issues that I had at home or to speak of the assault. Feeling like I had no one to turn to, I started writing poetry about the pain I refused to express out loud. While at school I found a love for Chorus class. I then decided I would write music about the hurt I was facing. It became my dream to be a voice for the kids who dealt with the same or similar struggles that I was going through.

During my senior year, I posted one of my poems on Facebook and someone saw it and asked how many more I had. She ended up getting a book of my poems published which is now available through many online retailers. We decided to release it to follow the dream I had to be that voice for those who might be going through similar situations.

As an adult, I had released music, made appearances on local TV, and been part of a pilot for a reality television series. Even with all of those successes, I still had faced depression. It never truly went away. Those hurdles, that voice in my head saying "you'll never be anything" still haunted me. It got to the point that one day, I put a gun to my head. I couldn't bring myself to pull the trigger though. The thought of the heartbreak my mom, aunt, and grandma would face if I was to actually take my own life stopped me. I laid the gun down. I curled up in a ball bawling on the kitchen floor.

The next day, my mom took me to talk to a counselor. After calling my friend Sharon, we all felt like the right thing to do was to check in at a behavioral health center. I felt as if I just needed to hit that "refresh button." While there, I met people who have been through way worse situations. It made me appreciate my life even if I had been dealt a really unfair hand of cards. It made me realize someone else is always going to have it worse than you.

I became friends with the people I met there. We talked about our darkest moments. We cried together. We also laughed together. Throughout the program, we became stronger together. We also wrote letters to each other. When I feel lonely or as if I'm at the end of my rope, I go back and I reread their kind words. It's amazing to see how in seven days I helped to change someone's life and how they did the same for me.

I can't express enough how much writing has helped me make it through my worst times and knowing that my words can reach people who may need it. It makes me want to work even harder on getting my poetry out to the right people. I wrote a little poem on day seven while waiting to be discharged from the behavioral health center:

Boy, your world has been brutalized.

You have been scrutinized.

It's time to rise above and shine.

You're about to take back your life.

I made a promise to myself that once I got out of there, I would take back my life and start making beautiful memories to cover up what has controlled my mind for so long. Finding the light after such a dark time felt like finding a pot of gold at the end of a rainbow. Once that sunlight hit, I found that freedom ... **my rainbow**.

To anyone in school who feels like ending their life over the words of bullies, I know kids and teenagers can be hateful. Once you are out in the real world, those name brand clothes and iced-out jewelry won't matter anymore. Real honest people are going to only look for genuine true hearts. Please, keep that beautiful personality and stay true to yourself because changing to fit in will only cause you to lose who you truly are. Turn your pain into art whether it be painting, singing or even writing. Don't let that pain build up inside and cause you to make a decision that will break hearts all around you.

I believe forgiveness is the key to moving on. Forgiving everyone and everything that has caused me pain has allowed room for me to become a stronger person. The best advice I can give to anyone who is going through depression daily or periodically is to never give up on yourself. Never allow the people who have hurt you to own you or run your life. To everyone else, please think before you speak because words live in the mind forever.

As of who Thomas Newman Powell is today, I am a better person. I have a relationship with both of my parents. I forgave them both for their mistakes. As far as my depression is concerned, I still have days that are harder than others, just like anybody else who deals with this disease of the mind. Some days you feel like going out to the ocean and watching the waves crash in and some days you can't bring yourself to get out of bed, and that's okay. It's okay to not be okay. Call someone. Reach out to those around you.

Remember that each day is a new chance at life.

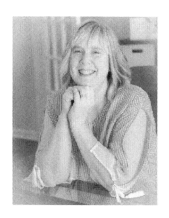

Cherie Faus-Smith

Keynote speaker, author, blogger, and transformational coach, Cherie Faus-Smith is a beacon for victims of domestic abuse. She shines a light on survivors and illuminates a path of prevention toward healthy relationships with an end goal of helping them recognize the signs of abuse.

During her journey of healing from abuse, she was diagnosed with panic disorder and in 2006, she became agoraphobic. Cherie shares her experiences to provide hope and inspiration to others.

Living her best life, she is spreading awareness about domestic abuse and mental illness. You can find out more about her at www.cheriefaus-smith.com.

Breaking Free

By Cherie-Faus Smith

"If nothing ever changed, there'd be no butterflies."

– Author unknown

The light turned green and I sat there paralyzed, unable to press the gas pedal. My young son sat in his car seat, oblivious to his mom's complete mental breakdown. As he stared out the window, I was trying to find the courage to move the car forward.

I felt instant fear. It was my responsibility to keep my child safe. But how could I do that without feeling completely out of control?

And then I heard his tiny voice, "Mommy, are you okay? The light is green. You can go."

The car behind us honked their horn, then did it again. My mind raced. The sweat on my palms made it difficult to keep my hands from slipping on the steering wheel. My knees shook but I still couldn't lift my wobbling leg from the brake.

I gave myself a pep talk. *"You can do this, Cherie.*

Your son is counting on you."

Slowly, my foot slid from the brake to the gas pedal and we were on our way again.

Looking back on my life, I always had a tad bit of anxiety but never fully felt the impact until my early twenties. I went through my school years with the normal nervousness of starting a new grade, not knowing who I would eat with at lunch or who would be in my class.

Once settled in, I was very outgoing. I had many friends and took part in many extracurricular activities. During band competitions, I was the first to step onto the field. It was a rush and I always felt proud of myself. In swim meets, softball games, and band competitions, I never once was nervous or felt anxiety. I was in my element.

If I was confident and full of life in my younger years, where did this anxiety come from? My parents told me that feeling nervous before a big event or a test was absolutely normal. As I aged, I would tell myself that the anxiety I was feeling was okay. But, was it?

Between the ages of 16 and 30, I experienced three abusive relationships. Each one was worse than the previous one. By the third relationship, my anxiety was at an all-time high.

Each morning when I awoke, I never knew if my

husband at the time would be in a good or bad mood.

I would automatically assume it would be a struggle and I would put my guard up.

In that relationship, I was in a constant state of fight or flight, and I truly believe that my body remained in that state of fear for years after we divorced. To be honest, I didn't fully deal with or heal from that trauma. I pretended it was over and gone.

Fast forward to my current life, my present husband and I will celebrate another year of marriage in August. He is kind, thoughtful and gentle - a true partner. But it hasn't always been roses and chocolates.

When we first met, almost 20 years ago, I put on quite the facade. You know, the one where our world is perfect, and we've experienced nothing bad in our life? I hid all my fears and smoothed all my stress so he wouldn't see them. We spoke every single day in the beginning of our relationship and I never felt more alive and excited than I did when we were together. He gave me hope and provided a safe space to share my life with him. He wasn't scared when I told him I had been married twice before and had a three-year-old son from my previous marriage. He accepted me for me, a welcome relief.

Shortly after we married, we tried to get pregnant. We wanted to experience the birth of a new life together and give my son a sibling. After a year of trying with no luck, we sought help from a fertility specialist, but the news wasn't in our favor. We decided that if it was meant for us to get pregnant, then it would happen. Yet, just a few months after that visit, I became pregnant.

I still remember that day as if it was yesterday. When I showed my husband the positive pregnancy test, he was in shock. He said he didn't know what to say. I expected him to hug me, to cry and shout "Hey, we're pregnant!" I didn't get that reaction at all. I'm sure he was just protecting his heart. The fertility specialist suggested that the odds of me carrying a pregnancy to full term was unlikely. I wanted more from my husband. I wanted him to pick me up, twirl me around, and say, "Babe, we did it! We're going to be parents!" despite the odds.

It wasn't meant to be. A few weeks later, I miscarried. We continued trying, but it never happened for us. My husband was okay with it because he loves my son as his own.

A few weeks after the miscarriage, I was lying in bed sound asleep when my son snuck into our bedroom and rocked me back and forth in bed until I woke up.

"What?" I yelled.

He replied quietly, "I had a bad dream mommy. Will you come sleep with me?"

For those of you who are parents, it's so much easier to give in and respond with a YES than to say no. If you say no, they will be back over and over again, until you give in to their request. It took enormous willpower to get up out of my warm bed. We walked to his room and I tucked him back in. As I lay beside him as he drifted off to sleep, I began to feel nauseous and anxious.

At first, I chalked it up to being startled awake, but those feelings got worse. Okay, I thought, maybe my blood sugar is low. So, I quietly crawled out of his bed and walked downstairs to grab a peppermint patty. I shoved it quickly into my mouth but as I tiptoed back up the stairs, my heart began racing.

"What is wrong with me?" I thought.

I ran into our bedroom and shook my husband awake. "Babe, something is wrong. I think I'm hemorrhaging from the miscarriage. You need to take me to the hospital to be checked out." He looked at me as if it was a bad dream and closed his eyes again. I shook him again and yelled, "Get up. We have to go!" But before he could walk too far, I collapsed onto the bed. The next thing I remember was this burly male about six feet tall taking my blood pressure. He looked at me and said, "Sweetheart, you are just fine. I think you had an anxiety attack."

"WHAT?!? You don't know what you're talking about,"

I replied scornfully. He glanced at his partner before turning back to me to repeat himself.

"Nope, you're wrong," I told him. "You need to load me into the ambulance and take me now."

"Your husband can take you if you really want to go.

There's no need for him to pay the ambulance fee for something that isn't an emergency," he responded respectfully.

But, that wasn't good enough for me and they ended up transporting me to the hospital. I can be quite persuasive and while I didn't know what a panic attack was, I was sure it couldn't be as bad as this.

After arriving at the hospital assuming they would take me in right away, I ended up waiting hours to be seen. Meanwhile, my husband and son fell asleep in the waiting room while watching SpongeBob SquarePants. That night is burned into my mind. My world turned upside down on the day that followed. A nurse called my name and three of us meandered back to a private room. She asked me to undress and don a fashionable gown with the tie in the back. I plopped myself onto the bed and she covered me with a sheet.

After asking multiple questions, she threaded the needle of an IV into my tiny veins. A warm and relaxing feeling overcame me. When I came to, the nurse was standing over top of me, confirming the news of my miscarriage. Okay, that wasn't really news to us but glad she felt the need to share.

She then looked at my husband and asked, "Is it possible for your wife to quit her job?"

Um ... we were a two-income family, so the answer was obviously no!

"May I ask why she would need to quit her job?" my husband wanted to know.

She quietly said, "I think she may be having a mental breakdown and she needs some time to rest at home."

"Well, if you think it's best, then obviously the answer is yes. I want what is best for her," my husband replied.

Because my body was being pumped full of some wildly relaxing drugs, I wasn't able to respond quickly enough before she exited the room. I didn't want to quit my job. I didn't want to feel like this. I didn't want to feel stuck. A few hours later, they released me. The drive home was eerily quiet.

We arrived home with the sun just coming up. I assumed my husband would stay at home with me after my frightening ordeal the night before, but he began to dress for a day in the office. I begged and pleaded with him to stay home with us. "I wish I could, but I have a big meeting today that I can't miss," he said. Life had to go on and he couldn't babysit me.

To be honest, I didn't want to be left home alone. I was afraid of what could happen. Would I have another panic attack? If I did, what would my son do? What would he think? I wasn't even sure I had the capability to take care of both of us.

Despite getting through that day, I woke up each morning thereafter with the same panic clawing at me.

The following year was hell. Not only was I suffering from anxiety attacks, but I also became agoraphobic. I avoided places or situations that might cause a panic attack or where I felt trapped. Being in a crowd or an open space was challenging. The fear became so overwhelming that I wasn't able to leave my home. The simple task of walking to the mailbox was out of the question for me.

I would stand at the door looking outside, wishing that I could walk outside to enjoy the fresh air. Another part of me, the irrational part of my brain, told me if I walked outside, I would float up into the sky. I'm also afraid of heights, so floating to the sky set my heart racing and shortened my breath too. Life as I knew it would be different.

My husband was very empathetic. I know I must have frustrated him, but he never showed that to me.

51

Because I could not leave the house, I missed out on my son's school activities. Talk about mom guilt! Luckily for me, those were my own feelings projecting - my son never made me feel different. He was fortunate, too, because my husband treated my son as his own and made sure that he filled the parental shoes until I could.

Being home alone during the day was tough. I was having five to six panic attacks a day. If my mom or a friend would call, I wouldn't talk long on the phone. My racing, irrational thoughts would trigger a panic attack. Days were long and the nights were even longer. I would wake up every night in a panic. My husband couldn't get a full night's sleep because I would wake him in the midst of a panic attack. Night after night, he stayed so calm, telling me, "You're going to be okay. Take deep breaths. I'm here for you," all while holding me.

I ordered a workbook on anxiety and agoraphobia but even reading my own symptoms caused a panic attack. I ordered a program that was specific to anxiety but after the first two audiotapes, I stopped listening. My life was at a standstill even though everybody else's lives were moving forward.

Nothing else was working so I turned to therapy. I had no idea how to get to the first appointment, though, since I couldn't drive myself and just leaving the house caused a panic attack. I had begun to hate car rides because anytime I left the house, my body would shake. My husband drove me to that first appointment. I clearly remember wearing my black boots with gray stirrup pants and a black leather jacket. I remember because my feet shook the entire twenty-minute ride and I held onto the side of the door, white-knuckling it the whole way there.

It took everything for me to sit through that forty-five-minute appointment. My palms were sweaty, I tapped my foot on the floor, and couldn't concentrate on what she was asking me. She explained that I was suffering from an anxiety disorder, which made me even more anxious. It was a never-ending cycle.

Despite being one of the hardest things I'd ever done, I continued on with those appointments. I gradually began to feel better, but it was a lot of hard work. It was definitely baby steps. In order to heal, I knew I had to push myself and I wasn't a quitter. I survived three abusive relationships. I was a fighter. I *am* a fighter.

While my husband was at work and my son was at school, I forced myself to step outside, even if it was for only fifteen seconds. Those fifteen seconds turned into thirty seconds and eventually into a minute. To keep my mind occupied during the day, I would rearrange our cupboards and go through our cans and throw anything out that had expired. I would clean the house and do the laundry in hopes that I would be too busy to have a panic attack. I began forcing myself to make phone calls and stay on the call for longer than a few minutes. My therapist suggested exercise would be good for me, but every time I stepped on our treadmill my heart rate would go up. My racing heart would trigger a panic attack because my mind would think that I was in the fight or flight mode.

I didn't give up, even though I had setbacks. I wanted to prove to my husband, and to myself, that I could be a good wife. I didn't want to miss out on any more of my son's events. We lived only a few miles from his school, and I wanted to be able to pick him up when the bell rang. That became one of my goals.

One day, I took a chair outside along with a journal and began writing my feelings. I no longer wanted anxiety and panic to run my life. I forced myself to stay outside even though I really, *really* wanted to run back inside. I refused to give in to those negative thoughts. My anxiety attacks began near the end of 2005. I still wasn't able to work outside the home at that time and I felt guilty for not providing an income for my family. So, in February 2007, I started my own company.

The only experience I had was as an administrative assistant. After researching the internet, I found there was a need for virtual assistants. It was new to me and I didn't know where to begin but I found a few clients along the way. It is twelve years later and I still own that company. I'm also an author, a speaker, and a mentor to women who have suffered domestic abuse.

I still live with anxiety and, on occasion, I still have panic attacks. Actually, a few years ago I became agoraphobic again after working so hard to beat It. I called my best friend one day and told her that I was having those horrible feelings again that made me afraid to leave the house.

Perhaps it came back because I work from home and I had no reason to leave the house. I only ever went out with my "safe person" - my husband. He loves me and because he loves me, he enabled me. If we decided to go shopping, and I began feeling uneasy, he would turn the car around because he didn't want me to feel uncomfortable.

When I told my friend of my fears, she told me that I beat it once before and I could do it again. When I talked to my husband about it, I told him the only way I would get better was for him to hold my hand, talk to me, and tell me that I could do it. I recognized that nobody could help me except me.

When I decided to write my memoir about surviving abusive relationships, I was working with a writing coach who knew about my anxiety and knew I was struggling. She told me after one of our coaching calls that I was to pick up my camera, get in the car, and drive somewhere and start taking pictures. It was something I love to do by being in nature. So that's exactly what I did. It helped me see that if I put my mind to something I could do it.

There were tiny accomplishments along the way. One day, I drove to the grocery store, which is about fifteen minutes from our home and had a list of three things that I needed to get. While driving there, I began to feel my anxiety creeping in. The negative thoughts, sweaty palms, the nauseous stomach. I thought I might pass out. But I made it to the store and after walking inside, I looked at the list and put those three items in my cart.

Once there, I called my husband and told him to guess where I was. He didn't know. I told him I was at the store. Knowing what a huge step that was for me, he told me how proud he was. Gone were the days where I hid my anxiety from him. He knew all of me and it put a smile on my face to know that he was there for me.

I still struggle with my emotions and I think I always will, but I refuse to allow my mental illness to dictate my life. I have a lot I want to accomplish, and I refuse to sit in my house like a prisoner.

Life is meant to be lived, and I'm going to live it.

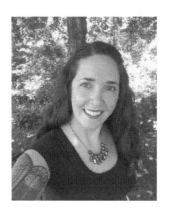

Holly Lynn Miller

While Holly Miller has eclectic passions, interests, and hobbies, she is easily summed up as a high school mathematics teacher who found a way to thrive despite her anxiety and depression. Her goal is to spread awareness about mental health, inspire those who struggle to see that they are not alone and show them that they can find light in even the darkest of places. She enjoys spending time with her husband Luke, their two dogs, two cats, and Russian tortoise. While she may not have many impressive credentials, Holly believes there is magic in the ordinary every day and that a simple life is a good life. She can be reached at
hollymiller1886@gmail.com.

Light in the Darkness

By Holly Lynn Miller

"The Light shines in the darkness, and the darkness has not overcome it."

– John 1: 5

There has always been something inside of me that I could not explain. At a young age, I would describe it as worry. Through my teen years, I called it stress. As an adult, I called it "being human" as a gesture at everything.

Being a contributing adult in society was soul-crushing to me, but I thought that was how everyone felt. Waking up every day, grooming, cooking, eating, going to work, grocery shopping, and interacting with people felt like an overwhelming burden by the time I reached my late twenties.

This darkness within me was something I tried to keep to myself. It was easier not to talk about it with others because it was so complex and I barely understood it. People who knew me as a young girl and people who know me today as a grown woman describe me as upbeat, motivated, caring, funny, and kind. Even my close friends would describe me the same way, possibly adding deep-thinking and maybe even a little tightly-wound if I let them inside my mind.

A friend recently told me she associates me with the word "bright" - happy, smart, smiling, helpful. No one understood the depths and complexity of the overwhelming dread I often felt. I believe myself to be an empath, absorbing others' energies, putting others' needs before my own, and often neglecting myself to make sure others have what they need. I am compelled to go to great lengths to make sure everyone I come across feels loved and safe.

People often described this as selfless and compassionate, but most did not see the toll it often took on my own wellness to the point where I could not take care of myself. No one knew this dark part of me that I was terrified of. I ignored it myself as much as I could. I was a hard-working student all through middle school and high school and took learning seriously. I was in many extra-curricular and held leadership roles in most of those activities. I volunteered in my community and church. I tried to be the best I could be in roles of daughter, sister, and friend. In all measures, I was a "good kid" and a great student.

I would smile a little when someone asked me what I wanted to be when I grew up, because I couldn't picture it. I wouldn't admit it at the time, but I was sure

I would be dead before I reached the age of 25 and I couldn't explain why I felt that way. At the end of high school, I earned an academic scholarship from a prestigious school and after four years in college, graduated with honors holding a mathematics degree and a teaching certificate. I was immediately offered a teaching job right out of college and started teaching high school math at the age of 21. All the while, I struggled with all of my might to keep this darkness I felt at bay.

I had all the trappings of success but I was frustrated that I couldn't enjoy it. After years of successful teaching, going on to earn a Master's degree, and getting married to the love of my life, I was hoping this darkness would eventually seep out of my life. But it only intensified. I was happy in every outright sense, but there was a numbness that slowly overtook my life.

After a particularly hard start to the school year in 2014, I left a very intense meeting at work with my head spinning and immediately passed out. This led to a long string of inexplicable illnesses. I started getting very tired. There would be days in which I would sleep 14 hours or more and I still could not function. The sun felt too bright and hurt my eyes. I felt like I was moving through molasses. I would sit down to grade papers and after struggling through one graded test, I realized in horror that a task that should have taken five minutes took me over an hour to complete.

Other times, I felt like I couldn't slow my body down. My heart would beat rapidly and I would break out in a cold sweat as I tried to catch up on errands and chores. I would run a fever of over 101 degrees. I would turn shades of green and white and get too dizzy to stand. I would hear a high-pitched ringing, see dark spots in my peripherals, and my chest felt constricted to the point I would gasp for breath.

These symptoms often lead to passing out or throwing up or both. And I was ravenous all the time. I would get extremely hungry I was willing to eat almost anything in sight. In a three-month time span, I missed 13 days of work due to these symptoms. I would be so worried about missing work that I forced myself to get up, but I would get sick on the way to work and have to call off. I would pass out in the parking lot if I was able to drag myself there. In less than a year's time, I gained over 60 pounds although I exercised and tried to make healthy food choices. I was so tired and hungry all the time. I went to many different sources to get answers. I had all kinds of tests done and no one could tell me for sure what was wrong. Worse yet, I kept getting sicker.

Luckily, I found a doctor who sat down with me, gathered all my test results, background, family history, and my own thoughts, and for once,

CORRECTLY diagnosed me. I was diagnosed with General Anxiety Disorder, Major Depressive Disorder, and Panic Disorder. The bouts of passing out and throwing up where I felt like my body could not slow down were panic attacks that stemmed from anxiety. Days where I felt like I physically didn't have the energy to get out of bed and I moved as if stuck in slow-motion were side effects of my depression.

For me, it was mostly biological and physical symptoms. I did not have harmful thoughts or suicidal tendencies. But I felt flat, empty, numb. I was not happy or sad. I felt nothing. The darkest thoughts were when I would wake up and be disappointed that I had to face another day. I didn't want to die, but I wanted to sleep forever. I would open my eyes each morning and feel an overwhelming terror that I had to face another day.

I had a hard time with my diagnosis at first. I couldn't believe it as I walked out of my doctor's office that day. On the way to my car, I was a little incredulous about it. I could admit that I had unhealthy self-talk where I heard myself saying "You're not good enough, you don't do enough, why can't you do A, B, or C ..." I knew I was physically unhealthy with all my symptoms, these bouts of fainting and nausea, and my uncontrollable weight gain. I reasoned with myself. "I have a great job, a wonderful, happy and healthy marriage, supportive family, and friends who care for me. I can pay all my bills, put food on the table, and I really can't ask for anything else! I'm not really even sad! What is wrong with me?! I need to snap out of this!" However, I knew I felt awful and the diagnosis explained it all.

In my car after my doctor's diagnosis, I called two people that I absolutely love and admire who also have had struggles with mental illness. I immediately burst into tears with them on the phone because I knew my doctor was right and I saw how hard they had to fight and I felt like I would never be able to stand up under these diagnoses. I remember saying I would never feel better. I would never get back on track. I couldn't be like them. I was not strong enough. Knowing I had two women in my corner helped, but my brain whispered, "You are going to be sick forever. You are never going to overcome this. I am a darkness you can never part from."

As I hung up the phone after talking to these women warriors, I realized it was the first time I cried in over a year. I was unsure of how I was going to get better, but I swore I would try with all I had in me to fight back. It was the first real feeling of hope I had in years. When I got home, my husband hugged me for a long time and told me he would help in whatever ways he could. He admitted he knew something was not right with me and I am so grateful he helped me to see doctors and specialists and pushed me to get the help I needed.

The years of 2014 and 2015 were intense. I started taking medication to help with my diagnosis. My doctor warned me it would make me feel worse at first but not to stop taking it. My physical symptoms ramped up for about a week. I would sweat through my clothes, but be so cold I couldn't feel my hands. There were still days I endured debilitating panic attacks. Sometimes my anxiety would be so high, I would scream in my car or sob in the shower because I was convinced I didn't know how to be a human being. There were days I still could not get out of bed. I would stand up, feel dizzy, and pass right back out.

Soon, the panic attacks went from daily to weekly to monthly. Soon, the numbness dissipated and I had more energy. I no longer wanted to sleep my free time away. Having answers, while they were ones I didn't like at first, helped me fight back.

I did research on techniques like grounding for anxiety. I forced myself to exercise more and only kept healthy foods at home as options to push back against symptoms of my depression. I remembered what activities used to make me happy and did those things, even if I wasn't feeling them at first.

My husband was my biggest supporter in getting better. If I would wake up wanting to call off of work, he would tell me I could handle it. He would help make me breakfast, help pick out an outfit, pack a lunch, and nudge me out of the door with an encouraging hug. I would text him when I felt overwhelmed during my day and he reassured me time after time that I would be ok. He would cook healthy dinners when I came home drained from existing and wanting to order food or go through the fast-food drive-through. And when I didn't feel right, even admitting it to him and having him listen to how I was feeling gave me the courage to continue to press on towards better health.

He gave me a mantra that helps me a lot. When I am feeling anxious or depressed, he will grab me by both shoulders, look me right in the eyes while gently rocking me saying "You GOT this!" and then pull me in for a long hug. Even if I can't believe I can get through the day, knowing he believes it about me helps me to at least try.

As I continued to heal, I found the more I acknowledged my anxiety and depression, the less power it had over me. I started being more open about it with close friends and family and eventually started posting about it on social media. So many wonderful people were supportive, but I am sad to say I had people in my life that could not or would not try to understand.

While it was hard for me to do, I distanced myself from those people who berated me for being lazy, selfish, and over-emotional. I unfriended those on social media who were purposefully unhelpful or were willfully ignorant. I found that many people related to me and would message me privately to share their own struggles. The more I posted, the more people seemed encouraged. They told tales of how they fought back or even how they felt seeing someone they love struggle with mental health issues.

I felt like I was taking power away from my illness by openly acknowledging it and inviting others to do the same. I found spreading awareness helped motivate me to continue to get better and work on my own mental health. I would post how I felt, show progress in my health, and share what helped and inspired me on my own journey in good mental health.

In the Spring of 2017, I spoke with a friend from work who was having similar struggles. She decided to complete the "Couch to 5K" running program and I vowed to be her running buddy despite my thoughts of "I hate running and I look stupid doing it." Also around the same time, I adopted a very young, very energetic, and very demanding border collie/lab mix.

Despite my past negative feelings toward running, I started the program with my dog and my friend. Due to my anxiety, I would do "practice runs'" on my own so when I met up with my friend, I wasn't holding her back. I was motivated to be a good running buddy for her and my dog was thrilled with all the running we were doing!

I remember telling my doctor at a check-up after I lost some weight that I started the program and she got so excited. She had suggested it to me in the past, but I felt like it was impossible for me to run and enjoy it, being over 260 pounds with anxiety and depression. I remember expressing that I felt selfish spending time on myself. My doctor looked me straight in the face and said, "If you don't take care of yourself, no one else is going to do it for you. Do you want to feel this way forever? Or even feel worse than you do now?!" That resonated with me, and I decided to make my own well-being a priority for the first time in my life. I carved out time each week to complete my runs and became more dedicated and consistent.

In the beginning, I was ashamed at my physical state and how hard running was for me, so I started completing my runs in a cemetery at dusk. I figured "I'm going faster than everyone here so that's a start!" Doing something I thought was impossible for me was the biggest way I fought back against my anxiety and depression.

The "Couch to 5K" program sets attainable goals in short runs that you complete every other day or once every three days to ease you into running. I went from being unable to run for 30 seconds to being able to run three miles without stopping in only two months. I will never forget feeling a panic attack coming on for the first time I had to run for a full minute and for some reason, I saw the ridiculousness of an overweight woman having a panic attack about running in a cemetery and I started laughing. It was the first time I fought a panic attack off!

Tackling the seemingly impossible task made me see I can do hard things, and it pushed my anxiety and depression right out of the picture. Running also helped with my physical health. I dropped 20 pounds in a couple of months with consistent running. I eventually lost over 50 pounds as I worked towards a healthier lifestyle.

Running gave me the confidence to tackle other difficult things in my life. After finishing each run, I was overwhelmed with gratitude and filled with a long-forgotten joy. I will never forget crossing the finish line of my first 5K. I had friends and family cheering for me as I rounded the last corner toward the finish line, but I could barely see them through my tears of triumph. I felt as if I were leaving my anxiety and depression in the dust behind me as I sprinted over the finish line. I remember thinking, "TAKE THAT MENTAL ILLNESS! YOU CAN'T STOP ME!" It was the first time I felt like I had my health, both mental and physical, back in my own hands.

Completing my first 5K was such a glorious moment, yet a small part of me knew one never truly "beats" these kinds of illnesses. Living with my illnesses for some time now, I know that I will have days I wake up and my brain has convinced me that I don't know how to be a human being. I know there will be days where I feel so beat-down and numb, that I won't be able to face the world. But I found ways to fight back. I have my tribe of friends and family who will always look out for me, listen to me when I am low, and celebrate with me in my triumphs.

I found that practicing gratitude every day is helpful as well. When I don't feel like running, I remind myself I GET to run. There are people who will never have the physical capabilities to run, so I run with them in mind and with gratitude in my heart. When I am dreading work, I am thankful for a teaching job that I love and I remind myself that despite what my brain tells me, I AM good at my job. I keep a folder of positive notes and emails from students, parents, and colleagues that I make myself read when I am feeling anxious about work. When I don't feel like eating healthy, I remind myself that I am privileged to afford healthy food and the ability to make it in my happy little kitchen. There are so many people who are stuck in the same darkness with which I am all too familiar. So many of them do not survive it. I am beyond blessed that I was guided toward a path of healing and have a wonderful support system in place with my loved ones. I have learned that sometimes, it's ok to not be ok. Most importantly, I learned that there is nothing wrong with living with mental illness. It affects more people than anyone realizes. I found that being open about it can inspire not only yourself but others who maybe won't or can't talk about their own struggles.

Above all, I recognize that there is a higher being, a powerful positive force, that has held me all along. I don't like discussing religion, especially with people I don't know, because of how isolating and divisive it can be, but there is no doubt in my mind that there is light and darkness in this world. I have seen evidence of both evil and good. I am of a Christian background so I frame my beliefs mostly in that lens but I don't get caught up who is "right" and who is "wrong" in terms of beliefs or religious sects.

Even as a young child, I have always been fascinated with the use of "light" and "dark" in the Bible. John 1: 5 says "The Light shines in the darkness, and the darkness has not overcome it." I feel this sums up my mental health struggle. The darkness will always be present. I will never be rid of it as long as I live, but there is a light that can never be extinguished and it shines into every corner of my darkest parts. Even if it is a small flame, it is brighter than all the darkness there is. For me, the Light that God provides can never go out. I cling to that notion fiercely.

For anyone who struggles with mental health or knows someone who struggles and wants to understand it better, I liken anxiety and depression to the common cold. It is something most of us will experience in our life. It may be a few days where you feel under the weather, or you may be the type of person who always seems to catch it. You can do things to stave it off like exercise, eating well, and going to a doctor, or talking with loved ones. But for some of us, we are still going to catch it - and that is ok. It's completely normal and valid to take time to get better.

No one faults anyone for taking time to get better from the common cold. It should be exactly the same for times when someone is struggling with the challenges of mental illness. They must be allowed time to get better. They must be allowed to do what helps them heal. There is no shame in the common cold. I feel no shame when I have a panic attack, or my anxiety is overwhelming and I feel like I forget how to be a human being, or when I start to feel myself slowing down into a depression. I acknowledge it, whether that be just to my husband or a friend or two, or whether I post about it on social media. I ask for time to heal. I do what I need to do to push through the challenges I face. When I come out on the other side, I celebrate it.

I hope that others see my story and feel hope. I am currently a thirty-something woman who holds a steady job and has healthy relationships despite having disorders. It is possible for me not only to exist but to thrive. I have been through darkness and I know I will encounter it again and again. It is a part of who I am. I know I also have love and light among the darkness.

The light can never be extinguished and will always shine through. I want people to see this darkness now. I want them to know it exists in me and how hard I often have to fight through it. I think there is darkness in each of us that calls out. By acknowledging it and showing my darkness to the world, I can also show my light. We all have struggles. Sometimes the darkness seems everlasting, but if you look for it, there is light also. You only need the smallest amount of light to find your way.

Let's talk about how both exist in each of us and use our own light together to make the world a brighter place.

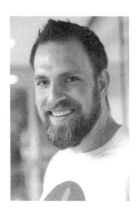

Justin Birckbichler

Justin Birckbichler is a men's health activist, testicular cancer survivor, and the founder of aBallsySenseofTumor.com. In November 2016, he was diagnosed with stage II testicular cancer at the age of 25. Throughout his diagnosis, surgery, chemotherapy, and being cleared in remission in March 2017, he has been passionate about sharing his story to spread awareness about testicular cancer, promote open conversation about men's health, and talk about the unspoken realities of being a cancer survivor.

In addition to his work through ABSOT, Justin's has written over 160 articles, appearing in Cure Magazine, I Had Cancer, The Mighty, The Good Men Project, Stupid Cancer, and more. His work with men's health awareness has been featured by over

60 different companies and organizations, including British GQ, Livestrong, Healthline, The Mayo Clinic, The Movember Foundation, National Foundation for Cancer Research, and various other groups.

In 2017, ABSOT won an award for the Best Advocacy and Awareness Cancer Blog in 2017 and Justin was recognized as one of 15 People Who Raised Cancer Awareness in 2017. Additionally, Justin was selected as the winner of the Hilarious Patient Leader Category in the 2018 WEGO Health Awards. In 2019, Justin was recognized as one of "40 Under 40 in Cancer."

Justin Birckbichler also serves as a member of the Strategic Advisory Board for the Cancer Knowledge Network, on the Board of Trustees of Our Odyssey, and on the 2019 WEGO Health Patient Leader Advisory Board. He also supports testicular cancer patients and survivors as the Testicular Cancer Hive Leader on HealthBeMe.

Outside of the "cancer world," Justin is an instructional technology coach, amateur chef, technology aficionado and avid reader. He lives in Fredericksburg, VA with his wife, cat, and dog. He enjoys reading, cooking, writing, exercise, and long walks on the beach.

Connect with him on Instagram (@aballsysen-seoftumor), on Twitter (@absotTC), on Facebook

(Facebook.com/ aballsysenseoftumor), on YouTube, or via email (justin@aballsysenseoftumor.com).

Ten Years Apart, But One Common Struggle

By Justin Birckbichler

"We don't make excuses; we make changes."

On my testicular cancer awareness blog, *A Ballsy Sense of Tumor*, I have written extensively about what it's like to experience depression as a cancer survivor. However, this wasn't the first - or even worst - time I have encountered a period of depression.

The first time I fought with clinical depression was ten years prior to my cancer diagnosis, during my sophomore and junior years of high school in 2006. For context, I grew up in an upper middle-class family. I am the oldest of three kids and my parents are still together. I was in the gifted program since third grade, took part in several sports, and school came rather easy to me. In essence, I was the definition of privilege and from the outside, I had no "reason" to be unhappy.

It all started gradually - almost slow enough that I didn't realize anything was amiss. Around the start of my sophomore year, I realized I was increasingly feeling sad and hopeless. Nothing seemed to bring me joy, and I always managed to find the negative in every situation. I couldn't figure out why this was happening, but I felt too ashamed to open up since I had a pretty good life. However, there was a lot of pain inside that I just didn't know how to manage.

I turned to self-harm to try to let out some of this pain. This is the first time I am publicly admitting this. Before writing this chapter, less than five people in the world knew I did this. I didn't want to cut myself since that would leave marks, which would make it hard to keep under wraps. I had done a stunt previously where I sprayed Axe body spray on my hand and lit it on fire. It didn't cause pain if you did it as a stunt, but if you let it burn long enough, it hurt like hell. I did this a handful of times. It didn't seem to help, yet it became a habit.

I suppose I subconsciously wanted to let some of this struggle out. I remember one day I put up an "Away Message" on AOL Instant Messenger that was beyond the scope of the normal, teenage angst. When I returned, one of my friends (who I later found out had depression himself) had said, "Um, Justin, you might be depressed." Even though I was self-harming from time to time, I didn't believe that I could be depressed. Again, I had a good life - what right did I have to be depressed?

At some point, this internal pain began to be too

much. I began thinking I just didn't want to live anymore since it was too hard, even though nothing external was "wrong." I started experiencing thoughts of suicide. While I never attempted it, I had concrete plans on how I would do it. It's still hard to walk past the area in my parents' home where I was planning to do it. My little sister ended up saving my life. She looks up to me and I didn't want to let her down. My love for her was stronger than my hate for myself.

Reaching this point was a pivotal moment. I finally admitted something was wrong, and I needed help. Yet, I didn't know how to ask. I stopped wearing a mask of being ok on the outside. I moved a little slower. I sighed a little more. I smiled less. One day, I flopped down dramatically on the couch and my mom finally asked if I wanted to talk to a therapist. Even though I was most likely weeks away from taking my life, I couldn't directly ask.

I agreed to get help and began seeing a therapist, Dr. S. I continued harming myself throughout the first few sessions and thoughts of suicide still lingered. Eventually, I admitted both of these to Dr. S and we agreed I would start on a course of antidepressants. Initially, we increased the dosage too fast and I experienced a panic attack not too long after beginning them. I freaked out because my mom told me to go to bed and I wasn't ready yet. I locked myself in my room and began hyperventilating. My dad literally kicked down my door and carried me outside to get fresh air. I calmed down, the doctors adjusted my meds, and the meds took hold.

I remember always being worried about my friends and other students judging me for taking medicine. Furthermore, I was even more anxious about people finding out I was going to weekly therapy. Being in high school and going to therapy weekly isn't exactly the easiest thing in the world to hide. I was constantly missing school for appointments, and eventually, my friends began asking me why I was never in class.

I usually said that I was seeing a doctor, but this ended up leading to more questions. After all, I didn't outwardly appear to be sick. I don't recall exactly, but I am sure I made up having various allergies and digestive problems to cover why I was frequently visiting a doctor. I would rather have people think I couldn't control my bowels than let them realize that I was getting help for my mental health. Looking back, that seems like kind of a crappy idea, but I didn't know any better.

It took a few more weeks, but a three-pronged approach helped me to begin feeling more like myself instead of an increasingly depressed teenager. First, the antidepressants helped get my brain's chemistry under control. Without these, I am not sure how long it would have taken for my mood regulation transmitters to get back in line, if that's even possible on its own.

However, the medicine by itself was not enough. Talking with my therapist helped me to control and change my negative thoughts. I suffered from major self-image issues and she helped me to reframe how I viewed myself so I could see the incredible young man that I was becoming. Though I never quite got past the self-inflicted "shame" of seeing a therapist, I took the various lessons that Dr. S. had taught me to heart and strived to truly embrace them daily.

The final, pivotal element of change came from a suggestion from Dr. S. I began exercising more. The American Psychological Association suggests that exercise can aid in treating and decreasing depression by helping the body's natural production of serotonin, along with helping to regulate sleep. I began running a few miles every day, and this led to me joining the track and cross-country teams, which helped my self-esteem and self-worth once I worked my way into varsity levels.

I honestly cannot point to just one of these three variables in helping me even out and alleviate my depression. They were a trio that helped save my life. As my depression improved, the frequency in which I needed to go to therapy decreased. I went from weekly visits to every other week, and finally settling into a pattern of monthly appointments. Both suicidal thoughts and desires to self-harm completely disappeared from my mind and I actually enjoyed living life.

After somewhere between twelve to eighteen months of therapy, antidepressants, and regular exercise, Dr. S, my pediatrician, and I felt that I had resumed my normal level of functioning. Because of this, my parents asked if I could get off of my medication and I agreed to try. Just as we had to taper on to the pills, I had to slowly decrease as I got off of them. To help mitigate any sort of unwanted negative effects from coming off of the pills, I went back to weekly therapy visits. To be honest, getting off of them was an uneventful process and I luckily avoided any panic attacks. Eventually, I was completely off of the meds and stopped going to therapy. I never experienced another depressive episode for the rest of high school and college and genuinely enjoyed life.

One final thing to note from this section of my life is that I rarely talked about this timeframe to anyone. I could count on one hand how many people knew about this experience as it was occurring. My very best friend never even knew about it. From the start, I had decided to keep this a secret and never planned on going public with my struggles. This experience was probably the hardest in my life. However, if we fast forward a decade, this trying period in my life ended up helping me recognize the symptoms early on during my survivorship phase of cancer.

I know that having depression at a young age puts me

at risk for a recurrence later in life. A 2017 study reported that about 20% of cancer survivors experience PTSD (Post Traumatic Stress Disorder) symptoms within six months of diagnosis. The CDC (Centers for Disease Control) also reports that cancer survivors take anxiety and depression medication at almost twice the rate of the general population.

At about a year of remission, I encountered various changes to my mood and personality. This included general feelings of "flatness," irritability and random outbursts of anger, difficulty sleeping, loss of interest in activities, moodiness, and many more signs that have come and gone throughout the past few months. These all came to a crux in October 2017 when I experienced a panic attack while watching one of my favorite Netflix shows, *Stranger Things*.

Finally, it dawned on me. I was experiencing many of those same initial feelings I had back in 2006. This time, not wanting it to get as bad as it did back then, I took a more proactive approach and decided that I would ask for help and antidepressants at my next doctor's appointment. Experiencing the episode in high school helped me advocate for myself earlier before it got worse.

In December 2017, I had my 18-month follow-up from my successful course of chemotherapy. After my oncologist told me that my scans were clear, I asked if I could go on antidepressants. I knew from previous experience that I respond well to these medicines and they helped balance me in 2006.

On my drive home, I asked myself, "Is taking these pills a cop-out?" Honestly, I didn't have an answer at the time. A few hours later, I was doing a Facebook Live video another cancer survivor, and I found my answer. The pills were not a cop-out. The pills would not be the only way I find happiness. Writing helps me process. The gym keeps me healthy, inside and out. These pills were just another tool in my toolbox for helping me to maintain a positive outlook, which is something I struggled with since the end of chemo. I wrote the following down as a reminder for myself:

"I'm not broken. I'm not weak. I'm not a lesser person for taking these. If I've ever felt brave along this journey, it's now. I'm asking for help and advocating for my own needs. It's a step in the right direction to putting me back onto a path of happiness."

You can't always tell if someone is experiencing depression from the outside. As I said, I had (and still have) a great life and no real reason to be upset. Depression is a chemical imbalance in your brain and it's always influenced by external factors.

Asking if a person is feeling okay won't always work, either. They might not even be aware of their own feelings or may hide it out of a certain feeling of stigma. My best advice to be there for that individual and to be non-judgemental. In 2019, we should be treating mental health as a serious issue and stop the stigma surrounding it.

Recently, I realized my mental health was again beginning to falter and I made the decision to begin seeing a therapist regularly. Though it's in the early stages, I know it will pay off. Even though I am very open about my mental health, I know that I can take even better care of it.

Though I kept my high school depression experience to myself, I've now taken a more public stance on sharing my struggles. I hope by sharing my story, even one person realizes that it's okay to ask for help and doesn't feel they need to suffer in silence. I compare taking care of mental health to needing chemo for cancer or a cast for a broken arm. No one would blink twice about treating either of those conditions, but why does society not have the same attitude towards mental health?

Furthermore, as a testicular cancer survivor and mental health advocate, I am especially passionate about opening up lines of dialogue in the men's health space. I'm closing with a challenge for all men reading this. Open up to one of your male friends about your mental health. Encourage them to do the same to you and to another friend. The tiniest ripple of one single conversation will eventually gain momentum and build to an overwhelming positive tsunami of change.

These conversations are definitely needed. The American Psychology Association reports that 9% of men have daily feelings of depression or anxiety and that over 30% of men have suffered from a period of depression at some point in their lives. These are just the statistics from men who responded to the survey and were honest with their feelings, so I am inclined to think the real numbers are even higher.

Change begins with us. As men, we can change this narrative and shape the conversation that it's ok to not be ok and it's totally cool to admit it. Share your own struggles or feel free to use my story as a springboard to get the dialogue flowing. The important thing is to have that conversation and keep it a constant part of life.

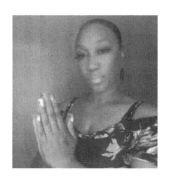

Nikki Burgess

Nikki B. is an inspiring entrepreneur and lifestyle influencer. She is a wife and mother, creating healthy and wealthy lifestyles. Her "Journey2-success" has become not only the attribute she offers as her brand, but also the goal she has set for her team, as well as herself. Besides growing her empire, she deeply enjoys spending time with her husband and children. She is currently a Financial Educator, helping everyday people have personal financial success by saving, keeping more of, making, and investing more money. She also encourages women to properly care for themselves in a major way. She is currently working on her autobiography, starting her own company and empowering women, men, boys, and girls to live their dream life. You can reach her at nburgess928@gmail.com, on Instagram @iamqueennikkib, and on Facebook at www.facebook.com/dreamnikki.

Mentally Unbroken

By Nikki Burgess

"Nothing is impossible. The word itself says, "I'M POSSIBLE."

– Audrey Hepburn

I had a very rough childhood. I often felt unwanted, displaced, and lost. Sometimes I would tell myself I was not where I should be - and this was at a very young age. Before my first birthday, 11 months to be exact, I bit into an electrical cord that was plugged into an outlet and I got electrocuted. I definitely know now that I'm truly supposed to be here and there's more for me.

I was a great student and I stayed out of trouble as much as I could. However, I remember being made fun of by my peers when I once shared an extremely traumatizing situation. I still enjoyed being in school and loved learning as I do now. Reading was my favorite subject and got teased a lot about being smart and was treated as if it was such a bad thing. I was called a nerd, a geek, and even a bookworm for being smart. How sad is that? Yet, the kids who made fun of me in school were the same ones asking for help and wanting me to do their work. Go figure! That always amazed me.

It was very difficult for me growing up with a mother who worked all the time, but I appreciate her beyond belief. I was the oldest and had to be a responsible child. I remember at the age of 14, I started telling myself that I needed more freedom to do what I wanted. I thought I could run my life. That was neither true nor healthy. All of these responsibilities made me grow up a lot faster than what is considered normal. I hung around a lot of older people, and I believe that also made me grow more rapidly.

Unfortunately, I started to get myself into trouble and I went from nerd to popular real quick. Again - go figure! I got into fights when some of the guys from school took a sudden interest in me and a lot of the young ladies in my class became jealous. I started defending myself for something that I had no control over and things that had nothing to do with me.

I pushed through as we often do when we struggle. I did the best I could every day and just pretended I was ok. I suppressed my feelings as if nothing was going on with me internally. I soon found myself in situations where I was being manipulated and taken advantage of often.

People did inappropriate things to me that caused dysfunction in my heart and mind. I started to numb any feelings related to those incidents to protect myself from the pain they brought. This behavior was detrimental to my mental and emotional wellness, and frankly life-threatening. I remember having that "I'm just going to go with the flow attitude," not really caring about how I'm doing, where I'm going, who I'm going with, or what I'm doing. None of that mattered to me at all. Living this way got me into situations and places that were what many would call unbelievable. I wish I would have just stayed at home some of those days rather than making those choices.

I've always been an outspoken, free-spirited woman and that's what has started many arguments over the years. I was just being myself and I felt like people couldn't relate to my personality. It's amazing how being yourself could cause so much pain from individuals that don't understand themselves and the actions that they carry out. Such people can cause a person to suffer and struggle, possibly their entire life.

Having access to anything I wanted was a concoction for disaster. Yet I still felt it was entertaining. Unfortunately, I became the entertainment while seeking attention from the opposite sex. Partaking in drinking and smoking became normal for me. To be perfectly honest, I didn't want to worry or care about anything or anyone but myself. That was life.

I shared none of my darkest secrets with anyone until

I got older when it was too late. Things that took place could have been avoided if I had shared sooner. Sadly, the things I inflicted upon myself were what I wanted to do and it gave me a sense of purpose - but unhealthily. It made me feel as if I was wanted and needed. Sometimes, you don't understand the severity of things until you come out of them and step back to think about what you've done or been through. We have to be aware of our surroundings and actions so we can be more receptive to our feelings and emotions.

I never thought I would face depression at the very young age of 14. As I stated before, my mother was a very hard-working woman and I had the responsibility of taking care of my two younger sisters: teaching, feeding, and protecting them. I will never forget one particular day when we lived in an apartment building in downtown Detroit, on the fifteenth floor. I was so angry because my mother allowed one of my younger sisters to used the "I'm the younger sibling card" to blame me for something that was not my fault. My mom immediately defended my sister for something that was not true. I was taking care of them the best I could and now I was being accused of something I didn't do. I was already struggling emotionally and this made it worse.

I broke down crying. I remember taking a pill bottle and pouring the entire bottle of pills in my hand. I looked at them carefully and quickly put them in my mouth and swallowed them. I had attempted suicide, and it is by the grace of God that I'm still here. That was not the only time I thought about ending my life. We know that things will happen in life, but when there are traumatic and life-threatening circumstances, it's hard to come out of those so we feel as though we need to take our own life and just end it all.

That day was the opening of my mental health challenges, and it all started at 14 years old. The pain (and resentment) of feeling defeated is the most unbearable feeling. It got harder because I didn't want to talk about what had happened. I was worried about what others would say, think, or feel about me after they found out I was struggling. I didn't know how they would look at me after finding out. I bottled up my feelings and tried to convince myself that the incident never happened. I did this until I later found myself in a similar situation and it took over every fiber of my being. I couldn't go on.

The good thing about the problems I faced as I was growing up is that I learned to face what was ailing me. I learned to stop and think about my decisions and how it would affect everyone that is a part of my life. The second time I was suicidal, I already had three children and thinking back to that very first dark period in my life helped me think about all of them. I thought about how I would leave them and how that would be selfish of me. I immediately got a sense of strength that allowed me to keep going another day.

Sadly, I endured more trauma again in my life. I got a heavy feeling of excruciating pain. I felt like there's absolutely nothing I could do. Nothing worked. I didn't enjoy taking medications so, unfortunately, I suffered through the pain.

One beautiful day in 2008, I was cooking breakfast, and I needed to go to the store to grab a few things. I remember one of my children asking if they could go and I said, "No, I'll be right back." The store was only five minutes away from our apartment. I was walking down the street and when I got to the traffic light, there was no traffic. I remember looking at my left and I could hear a siren coming. It passed by me, but I waited. I could see down the hill and an ambulance was coming, so I waited patiently for it to pass by. There was a car stopped at the traffic light and when I crossed the street, it hit me on the left - BAM! That was one of the three most terrifying events that have ever happened to me. It was so sudden, yet I remember it like it was yesterday.

I looked up after hitting the ground and my fingers were sliding down the hood of the car. It was horrific. When I realized what had just happened, all I could say was, " why did you hit me?" People were driving by and stopping in the middle of traffic. It was one of the most devastating things that have ever happened to me. Sadly, I've had a lot more terrifying incidents in my life as I have described.

When that car accident happened, I was only 22 years old with two children. It was two days before my 23rd birthday. The EMT and police officers asked me if I wanted anyone to be notified. I asked them to call my fiancé who is now my amazing husband of seven years. He ran down the street but by the time he got down there, I was already in the ambulance and on my way to the hospital.

Since that day forward, I have had excruciating pain. There were days where I couldn't get out of bed. I was bedridden for months. I had a sling on my left arm. I had knee damage, neck and lower back disc herniation, shoulder nerve damage, and all these ailments caused me to be temporarily paralyzed. It was so hard for my family to see me in this condition and my husband was furious.

I believe everything in our lives happens for a reason. Today I can truly say that I am healed. I went through all of this physical and emotional pain, but that was the process for me to be here today and share it with others. I hope that anyone who has similar situations would know that there is a light at the end of the tunnel and that's where better and greater things happen. The power is in your mind and what you think. If you want to be healed, if you want to be something in this world and become the greater version of yourself, it all starts with your mind.

I am in a very happy place and my mission moving forward is to help at least one person to have faith, joy, peace, and happiness in their hearts and lives every single day. These gifts cannot be taken, but you have to work on your personal development daily. I practice deep breathing to stay well. Thoughts of suicide are utterly indescribable and I would never wish that on anyone, not even my worst enemy.

The golden dreams that I have right now for the future are simple. I just want to be the best version of myself so I can help every single person I encounter in this lifetime. I am considering becoming a spiritual life consultant to help people with every aspect of life including but not limited to business, parenting, finances, friendships, and marriage. I've been through a lot and I want to provide value while giving people a glimpse of hope. I want to help them grow and focus on what's important. I've always been a go-to person for people and that helps me understand that I have been through a lot and that I am here on this Earth to share my story. I am not saying this to put myself on a pedestal, but this is my gift and it's humbling to be living my purpose. Every day that I'm given breath, I plan to live on purpose.

Helping others maintain their mental health is very important to me. I want to help people stay positive through their struggles. Some days, this can be hard but we have to find moments where we can focus on what matters. I make time to take complete breaks from the stressors of life. I turn off social media notifications. During my mental breaks, I turn the ringer off my phone or only use my phone to interact with my husband and my children.

It is okay to cut off the entire world when you need to because if you're not healthy in every way possible, you will fall apart and you won't be there for those who depend on you. You can't be there for anyone if you can't be there for yourself. If you're constantly going nonstop, you will not have the opportunity to pause, reflect, energize yourself, and come back rejuvenated and ready to accomplish, conquer, and dominate everything that you touch.

I also affirm myself daily and that helps me maintain my mental health. Here are just a few words that I speak out loud on a daily basis as part of my daily affirmations:

I love and not hate.

I speak in respect and positivity or I say nothing at all.

If I choose to speak, I will speak the truth and nothing less.

I have the courage to live my dreams.

I am strong.

I am kind.

I am beautiful.

I am smart.

I am important.

I am Fearless.

I am amazing.

I have an overflow of supreme abundance.

I illuminate peace love joy & happiness that has been bestowed upon me from the Heavenly realm. My time is now.

This is my journey to success, and this is a glimpse of my story. I will always strive to be great, do my very best, and I will make sure I help someone else in the process. A lot of the things I experienced growing up made me the person I am today. I'm stronger having gone through those things so I could be here to share. We all face issues in life. We never know what it's for or why it happened. Early on, I always knew in the back of my mind that there was something better for me, but I did not understand what that meant or what that entailed until right now, at this very moment.

We should always remember that no matter what we face, our test becomes our testimony.

MADE TO OVERCOME

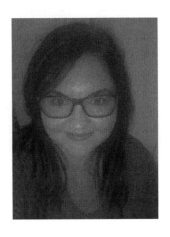

Dani Adams

Dani Adams resides in central PA with her son, Josiah. She enjoys using her gift of music and sharing her story to see others set free and walking in their true identity as sons and daughters. Dani is currently a first-year student at Global Celebration School of Supernatural Ministry (GCSSM), where she is excited to dive deeper into the love of the Father and going after all that He has for her. She is a member of the worship team at Movement Outreach. She enjoys her joy-filled moments with her son and living out loud together to cause Heaven and Earth to collide and spread joy everywhere they go. Dani can be reached at
DANI.adams8713@gmail.com.

My Journey

By Dani Adams

"Look with wonder at the depth of the Father's marvelous love that he has lavished on us! He has called us and made us his very own beloved children".

– I John 3:1 TPT

I do not remember life before depression. I am sure there were good moments with my family. Before my parents separated, we went on family vacations and to this day, the beach is still my favorite place to be. I am at the beach right now writing this!

My challenges started at a very young age. By the time I reached high school, I was on antidepressants, skipped half of the tenth grade and had to do correspondence classes via mail in order to graduate during the summer of 2005, instead of walking the stage with my class.

I grew up in a very religious home and my family loved as best as they knew how. They did not know what they did not know. There was a lot of dysfunction and abusive behaviors that came from multiple people in my life from a young age until it became an addiction. If someone was not abusing me, I looked for that because I knew nothing else. I did not know I was worth anything more.

My life became one of extreme isolation. I remember my mom begging me to go to a family function or go out to eat. I preferred hiding in my room. There was such turmoil in my mind from a young age. Suicide was a constant torment in my mind. So many lies took root as a little girl. I believed I was a mistake, that I was a nobody and my life could never turn around and make any sense.

When it came to those who surrounded me, some walked away completely and others I feel did care, but they did not know how to help. I only knew how to push people away.

I desperately wanted relationships and community, but I was so tired of being hurt. While in the moment of believing I am not worth anything more, I felt like I was stuck between a rock and a hard place. I wanted community, but I felt paralyzed by fear. I would lie about going to school and would hide in my room, or go hide in the woods. I let the lies of what people had said to me and about me, and the torment from the experiences cause me to feel trapped.

I had two pivotal points in my journey. The first moment was when I was 17. I was a senior in high school. I remember it as if it was yesterday. It was September 1, 2004. It was at about 11 p.m. I found myself in my bathroom at my mother's house and had plans to end my life that night.

As soon as I started to take action towards my plan, the presence of Jesus flooded the room. I grew up in church, but I had no idea that I could know my Heavenly Father personally. I never knew that Jesus wanted to be my friend. I knew nothing about the Holy Spirit, let alone the comfort He wanted to bring into my heart and life. I knew about God, but I never truly knew Him. I also loved singing in church and being involved. I enjoyed reading my Bible when no one was looking, but honestly, it was a bit confusing because I felt what I read contradicted what I heard in church on Sunday.

But that night, I felt the presence of Lord flood that bathroom. I heard the Lord invite me to take His hand. He promised to help me out of the pit I found myself in and it would be better than I could ever dream or imagine. In my heart of hearts, I did not want to truly end my life, but I did want out of the misery I was in. I felt stuck and I didn't know what to do. After I gave my yes to Jesus, I went to sleep and had a dream about the plans and the purposes that the Lord had for me. I had searched all over to find any purpose in life. I found that my only hope and help was in the name of Jesus.

Fifteen years later, I found myself in the same hole, but much deeper. I had switched churches where I was involved in a youth group on Wednesday nights and joined a worship team. I felt most alive in His presence and spreading the joy of the Lord to others. I worked very hard during my senior year of high school to graduate high school that summer. I ended up attending Bible college in Ohio and studying music. I was living my dream. Father had set me free from depression and all the torture in my mind. I was leading music for a women's Bible study. I really felt this was a new season.

While I experienced some deliverance in Ohio, I still did not know how deep the Father's love for me was. I lived in such condemnation and was sinking in shame. As I said earlier, I was addicted to dysfunction and abuse. Before long, I found myself in a relationship with a very abusive man that soon I would marry. We were only married for three months before I became pregnant. Once that happened, a light bulb went off in me. I started to understand that this innocent, unborn child deserved so much better. The relationship ended a little after that.

Fast forward to last summer when my son was seven, I learned of some abuse that my son had experienced from a family member. I was at the lowest place I have ever been. It was a constant battle between really not wanting to live another day, but I knew my son needed me and I had to keep fighting. I had to keep pushing. I had to keep going. Everything was at an all-time high. Once I found out what my son had walked through and I didn't even know it, I knew that I had to find a way out. I grabbed some of our clothes and drove away.

I knew that was it. I had enabled behavior in my family for far too long. I had walked on eggshells while I was dying on the inside. I really felt like the walking dead. I was bleeding to death from the inside. Within five days of leaving my father's house, my son and I were blessed with an apartment. I knew that this was the moment that I had to start over. It was time to get real. It was time to get honest. It was time to really search inwardly and be honest with myself about where I was at. Where I am is ok. I am safe where I am. Walking in awareness of where I am and where I truly want to be is so powerful.

Walking in gratitude was what I used to get from where I was to where I am now. I started to thank the fear of being here. I started to thank depression for being here. I started to thank different things in my life for being here. In walking in gratitude, I could let go and what I wanted started coming towards me.

What I didn't realize is that Heavenly Father's goodness and love were always flowing towards me, but I would often only allow His love to come to a certain distance. I was pushing away what I wanted and not even realizing it. Understanding that I am not trying to become something or someone else, I had to come to an awareness of who I already was.

I wasn't trying to chase success. I am already a success. I could live from the success that I already am. The more I focused on the truth, the more the torment would leave. Whatever I would focus on, I would have more of it. Instead of focusing on how terrible of a single mom I am and how my son deserves better because I could never be enough, I turned around and told myself how amazing I am, how I am enough, and how I am a really great mom. When I would feed the lie that I am not good enough, I would get just that feeling that I am not enough.

Another addiction I had since I was very young, was the addiction to food. It truly became my drug of choice. I believed that if I was fat and ugly, that no one would want me. Everyone would leave me alone. Deep down, I was starving for love and affection, and I wanted to be wanted, but the lies kept telling me that I was not worth anything. I'm just a trash can. I'm just a mistake.

One thing that has really helped with my mood is getting myself off the couch, and get up and get moving more. Instead of wanting to take naps all the time, I want to do fun things with my son. Getting my daily miles in from walking is something I really look forward to. I'm learning what it means to be kind to myself and to love myself. I'm also learning to experience and encounter the Father's love, to receive it for myself, so that I can share it with my son and with everyone around me. This world needs to be loved.

Having self-awareness and being grateful has totally shifted everything in my life - moving me from victim mode to being victorious. As a single mom, I would live this life of a pity party, saying to myself: "I'm all alone. I'm doing this all by myself." There is some truth to this, but I'm learning that I have a Heavenly Father who loves me so much, who wants to be there for me and wants to take care of every detail in my life.

Goodness is flowing towards me. When I tap into that flow, I experience more. Everything I have always wanted has always been available to me. The question is, am I open to what is available, or am I ok staying where I am? The truth is, I am not stuck. Everything is a choice. I am powerful enough and strong enough and brave enough and bold enough to make a decision and create the life I want to live. I never wanted to keep living. So what can I do about that? How can I rewrite my story? My past does not have to be my story any longer.

By the time you are reading this, I will have started my first year of classes at a local ministry school. I want my identity to be rooted and grounded in the love of my Heavenly Father. I'm no longer pushing away what I truly want, not just for me, not just for my family, not just for my son, but so that everyone that I come in contact with can experience that same love.

As I'm writing this, I am visiting my friends' beach house, and the memories I get to make with my son brings tears to my eyes. I want to make new memories, experience new things, just like my son told me. He said, "Mom, you need to try new things."

I absolutely love sharing my story and encouraging others. If Jesus can pull me out, He can do the same for them. The same love, joy, and victory that was available to me in my time of need, it is available to anyone and everyone. No one is left behind. No one is left out. There is a seat at the table for every single person reading this.|

To anyone that might be struggling, I want you to know that you are not alone. You are loved. You matter. You have a divine purpose and everything is going to be ok. You are brave enough and bold enough to make the choices you need to make in order to create the life of your dreams. You are worth it.

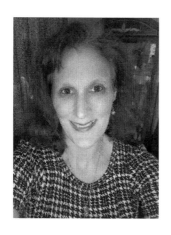

Shawnee Penkacik

Shawnee Penkacik is an author, social media manager, and podcast host. Her website Sunshiny Thoughts along with her podcast seeks to encourage moms to know their worth in Christ. She wants moms to know that although motherhood is messy and hard, God will give them the tools to make it through. Shawnee is married to her husband Jason of 22 years. When she is not juggling the duties of raising their eleven children, she enjoys her morning coffee, time with her family, or reading a good book.

Follow her on Instagram.com/sunshinythoughts to learn more.

Worry and Anxiety

By Shawnee Penkacik

"Do not be anxious about anything, but in every situation, by prayer and petition, with thanksgiving, present your requests to God. And the peace of God, which transcends all understanding will guard your hearts and minds in Christ Jesus."

– Philippians 4:6

Have you ever found yourself up late at night with a thousand thoughts running through your head? You know you need to go to sleep because you have a very busy day ahead but you can't. Maybe you have children and you need to be up to take them to school, but at the end of the night, you think about the events of the day. You repeatedly play those events in your head. What if this or that happens, or what if this person does this or that? You lay awake trying to prepare for every worst-case scenario but most of them never happen.

I settled into bed at night and a thousand thoughts would hit me like a plague. I would stress over appointments, my husband's job, whether so and so thought I was a good enough mom, whether I would walk that day, etc. It seemed only at night time, my worries and fears would get the best of me.

I remember one night, in particular, my husband was away on a business trip. I knew that I was the parent who was in charge of the kids the next day and that I needed sleep. But as my head touched the pillow, fear crept in like a wave washing over me like a flood. The kids were nestled in bed and sound asleep yet I ran around the house turning every light in the house to make sure no one would break-in. I turned on the music. I turned on the TV. I called a friend and stayed up late watching television, reading books, and working on the internet. What happened? Nothing. We were safe, and I had wasted an entire night of sleep.

The next day, I was exhausted. I had six children under the age of six. I had to teach three of them as they were homeschooled and I had a newborn to take care of. My husband came home from his trip the next day. I was so glad to see him. I hugged him and he knew that I had stayed up. He knew my fears had gotten the best of me. "Honey, you need sleep," he said.

I just needed that peace of mind with him in the house. It would continue every time he would go away on business trips, which took a toll on our relationship.

He knew that when he would announce that he had to go for a convention, regional meetings, etc, that I would guilt him and make him feel bad for leaving me when really I was just scared.

Worry continued to plague me. Especially when we moved to tornado alley. Now, I have asked God to not move us to certain places when my husband's job asked for us to relocate. Every time, we were sent us to the place that I said that I didn't want to go. One of those places was Tulsa, Oklahoma.

I loved Tulsa as it was the hub for the Bible belt with great churches but I hated Tulsa for the weather. We had a lot of good things going for us when we moved to Tulsa. We had a beautiful home to live in, a big backyard, and activities for the boys to be involved in. Our boys wanted to join sports when we moved to Tulsa. So my husband decided that they could play Tball.

I had heard about tornadoes like the ones in *The Wizard of Oz* but had never seen one in person. One night my husband came home early from work, our boys had a T-ball game. We were all excited to watch them play. In the middle of the game, the announcer came on and told us that the game was canceled because of a tornado warning. We gathered our boys and headed home. We stopped at Walmart and grabbed a few things for dinner. While we were in Walmart, the tornado siren went off. It sounded like a

111

freight train whistle, yet louder.

Suddenly, we were asked by an employee, if we wanted to go to the back of the store and take cover or head home to wait out the storm. If we left, we were responsible for what happened to us. We headed home as we had other children at home who we knew would be frightened. When we got home, I started to pray and gather supplies. I was in a full-blown panic mode. What would happen if the tornado hit the house? What was the probability of the tornado hitting the house? How could I make sure the children were safe?

I grabbed mattresses, called friends to inform them. My husband sat down in the living room, calm and collected. It made me mad that he wasn't taking it seriously. He told me to trust in the Lord, He would protect us. I continued to run around for the next half hour figuring out the storm or trying to. I was mad at my husband for not helping. He said, "I'll take cover when we need to and continued to sit in his chair." The storm passed over us and he was right. God protected our family. In fact, the whole time we lived in tornado alley, God watched over us. We would hear of storms hitting after we left and were in awe of the goodness of the Lord.

The fear of the weather is one thing that has now been passed down to my kids, especially one son in particular. He hates when storms are coming. He

112

tracks them on his phone or on the computer and goes outside to check the sky. The closest thing we had come to us in Arizona was a flood. In Colorado, he asked our neighbors if they get tornadoes, when was the last time one hit, and what he needed to do to prepare. He also asked his teachers, my friends, etc. He had a tornado bag that he kept under his bed that he would grab and head to the downstairs bathroom if he even had an inkling of a tornado within an hour distance.

One summer, he was at the part with his youngest brother. They were playing and being silly. Suddenly the sky started to turn green. We don't get storms like that in Pennsylvania, or so I thought. The winds started to rise and things started blowing. Both boys ran into the house with the screen door slamming behind them. I got them into the house and saw that same full-blown panic on my son's face. "I'm going to the basement, mom," he said. This time, I remained calm. I told him how we don't get storms as we had experienced in other states and that we would be safe. I prayed and my son continued to watch the storm as the rain pounded down and the winds blew. We lost briefly lost power that day and were not prepared. More panic went over my son and I'll admit it frightened me. However, when the clouds cleared up, and the rain stopped, we were safe. There were trees and wires that were knocked down by the storm, but our house stood strong. This changed the kids' outlook on playing outside when it would rain.

Maybe your worry isn't protection or weather-related.

Maybe your worry is about finances and whether you'll have food for the next day. I had many worries when we moved to Arizona. My health was up and down still and we had two boys who had feeding tubes and needed constant medical care. I worried about finding new doctors who would take care of them. Yet again God provided, and we met some of the best medical team doctors in Phoenix.

Finances became a worry when my husband lost his job after we moved to Arizona. We left our home in Washington because we were making countless trips to Seattle for medical care for our two boys. An opportunity arose for my husband to be a general manager in Phoenix. We prayed over it and decided it was the best direction to take. In a month of time, we bought a house which was the perfect price for us. However, after six months, the bottom started to fall out. Worry plagued both my husband and myself. We knew that God had led us to Arizona as he had directed the path for us to move. My husband was told the company was going in another direction and would no longer need him to manage the hotel. We sat there with a newly purchased a home, a car to pay and children to feed, wondering what would happen next. It hit me we could lose everything. I started to think about going back to work, selling things, and things I could do to take care of our family. However, in the middle of this, we had two sick children. We had one son who wasn't growing and needed constant medical care. Then another son was struggling again with his illness after being stable for years.

Turning Point

I was taught as a Christian growing up in the church that worry was a sin. Why was I struggling so much with worry? Maybe it was because I didn't know how to trust. People in my life had hurt me and let down more times than I cared to count. Trusting was hard for me. While I trusted God for my salvation, I felt that He had better things to do than care about the little things in my life. I am so glad that this changed. I started to dive deeper into my Bible. I read verses about how God takes care of the birds and how he clothes them in splendor. I traveled to the verses in the Bible about how God would supply all my needs according to His riches in Christ Jesus. However, when I was worried. I would run to the phone to talk to a friend. I would ask them to pray and talk about my struggle. In time, this changed.

I began to realize that God had given me the same authority that He had given my friend. I could pray the same way my mentor could, the same way my pastor could, and realized that God would hear me too. Then I watched as God did just that. He opened the door

115

for my husband to attend culinary school as a chef, a passion that he had since the boys were young. He provided for us with food to eat, with unemployment for a period, and we watched as miracle after miracle happened in our rough season.

I wasn't just worried about the weather, safety, and finances. I was also worried about my marriage, my friendships, my job, and whether people liked me. My worries were overboard. Then, one day finally realized that I was worrying too much. I wanted to win the battle over worry. I knew the scriptures in the Bible that talked about worry. One of them is found in Philippians 4:6 - "Do not be anxious about anything, but in every situation, by prayer and petition, with thanksgiving, present your requests to god. And the peace of God, which transcends all understanding will guard your hearts and minds in Christ Jesus."

Do not be anxious. God didn't want me to worry about whether we would have a home, or if the weather would take us out, whether death would darken my door. He wanted me to TRUST Him. He has a great plan for my life. I needed to remember that. Yes, bad things happen to good people. I know that. However, nothing had ever passed through God's hands that He didn't know would happen in my life. I would be okay.

Worry still hits me like a ton of bricks, especially for my children. But was that worrying adding a single day to my life? The answer is no. When you worry, you become stressed out and you lose sleep. Worry can cause headaches and make health problems worse. No wonder God tells us not to worry. The opposite of worry is trust. It is easy as human beings to want to know what will happen. We want to be secure, safe and feel loved. What was worrying doing? It was ruining my relationship with my husband, my children, and my friends. It was keeping me up at night and causing my health to get worse.

I dealt with worry again when I found out I was pregnant with my youngest daughter. The doctor told me because it had taken so long to get insurance and get things in place, that she may have some difficulties. They were sure she might have a rare disease or be born with delayed development. I started to wonder. Will she be like have eosinophilic esophagitis like her brother? Will she have seizures like her sister? Or could it be worse?

I was blessed to have my wonderful conference friends and Christian family pray over her. My health got worse as the conference approached and I found myself in the hospital. I needed a transfusion. My iron was drastically low. I had fallen and my health was declining. The thoughts plagued me again. Was I going to be okay?

As the worry hit, I started to pray: "God, I know you have a plan for my life. I know you gave us this daughter and you have a good plan for her. Thank

117

you, Jesus, for making her healthy and whole. Thank you for making her lungs work and be strong. Thank you for making her heartbeat as it should. Amen."

It was a short simple prayer. Jesus had us. I knew our daughter was a gift from God. I knew that even if she was born with challenges, God would yet again see us through. I prayed over her little life.

When we went for our next ultrasound, we saw a perfectly HEALTHY baby girl. She had ten fingers, ten toes, a beating strong heart, developing stomach, etc. I was so relieved. My team of doctors continued to monitor her and every time the result was the same. I'd write in my journal to tell her to grow healthy and strong. My health challenges didn't change. However, my faith grew stronger in that season. I had surrounded myself with strong Christian women rooted in their faith who would pray, who would read scripture, who would lift me up when I was down. I am pleased to say we welcomed our beautiful daughter in April 2019 and she was born 100% healthy. God had done a miracle in her and in me.

Coping skills are important when you struggle with worry and anxiety.

Coping skills - things you can do to help you calm down when you are anxious or worried - are key when you struggle with worry.

What can you do when you worry? For me, I can pray.

118

I talk to God about my worries and the situation I am dealing with at the time.

You can listen to music. Music is such a calming factor for me. I will listen to some worship or even contemporary Christian music and I am energized and ready to face what's ahead.

You can take a bubble bath or a shower. I love bath bombs so I use those infused with essential oils when I am stressed.

I journal when I am plagued with worry. I grab my journal and get all my thoughts on paper, even if they sound dumb. I put them on paper and sometimes I will tear the paper up and throw it away afterwards. I feel better because it has gone from my brain to paper. It's a brain dump exercise.

Take a walk. Getting alone with God and nature helps and the change of scenery often helps me see things from a different perspective.

These are some coping skills that I use. Yours will probably be different. My boys play video games to relieve stress. My husband will watch a movie.

You can win the battle over worry and anxiety. Just take it one day, and one step at a time!

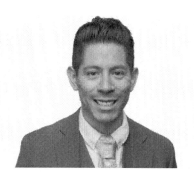

Dan Esterly

Dan Esterly was born in Tegucigalpa, Honduras and raised in Pittsburgh, Pennsylvania. Dan is an entrepreneur and has owned a consulting venture for the past three years. Dan obtained a Master of Business Administration from the University of Saint Mary and a Master of Science in Professional Counseling from Carlow University. He currently acts as Vice Chairman of the Board of Directors for Glade Run Foundation, Board of Directors for the Pittsburgh Project, and serves on an advisory committee for Global Links. In his spare time, he is an avid coin collector and art enthusiast.Learn more about Dan at www.danesterly.com

The Road Not Taken: A Story of Resiliency

By Dan Esterly

"You are not a drop in the ocean. You are an entire ocean in a drop"

– Rumi

In behavioral science, the past is often the best indicator of future behavior. While that concept remains true; I also believe that we are not defined by our past. In my experience, people are resilient, highly adaptable, and designed to confront adversity. The obstacles that life throws at us can seem unmanageable and the mountain too high to climb. Yet without those steep terrains, there would be nowhere further to reach and no breath-taking view from the top. This is my story of overcoming adversity related to mental health.

I was born in Tegucigalpa, Honduras in 1990. I was given a two-day life expectancy, because of starvation and malnourishment. I hit the life lottery when two amazing people from Pittsburgh, PA adopted and raised me. I had a great childhood by all accounts. I

121

didn't notice my depression until about age 10. I still remember expressing thoughts to my friends that seemed normal to me, but completely abnormal to them.

These were the earliest depressive thoughts that I can remember having. They often went something like "my friends would be better off without me," "no one likes me," or something along the lines of "'you don't belong here." Looking back, I don't think any one thing contributed to the development of my depression. It's something that I've spent a lot of time thinking about. I can tell you that my adoption affected me earlier in life.

I looked nothing like my family or most of the people I grew up around. I remember some occasions where people would stare at us in public. I also remember being asked a few times why I looked different. While there was no bad intention in either of these situations, it only added to my feelings of being different and not belonging. I didn't fully accept or make peace with my adoption until early adulthood.

There were other childhood events that I imagine contributed to the start of my depression. I endured sexual abuse over the span of a few years prior to my depressive thoughts developing, which I won't go into detail about within this chapter. However, I believe it created feelings of guilt, isolation, and poor selfesteem. I also experienced the first loss of a loved one during this time. Add into the picture the changes of moving from childhood into adolescence, my unknown genetics, and you could probably see just how many factors could have contributed to it.

I eventually received diagnoses of Major Depressive Disorder (MDD), Post Traumatic Stress Disorder (PTSD), and generalized anxiety symptoms that went along with them. It was very hard to figure out how to cope with these symptoms when I was growing up because I really did not understand what was going on with me. I got bullied as a teen for looking different and acting out because of what I was going through. This added to my feelings of being different and disengagement with school and peers. I earned average to below-average grades in school.

I had mentally tuned out and really didn't believe that I'd amount to anything in life. I would get into minor trouble at school, but never anything too serious. I eventually left public school and sought alternative forms of schooling that could accommodate my diminishing performance at school. I ended up finishing high school online through PA Cyber Charter School. This turned out to be the best decision that my family made because it allowed me to take dual high school/college credit courses at a local university.

I began college part-time at age 16 and was attending full-time at age 17. This was when I was first introduced to alcohol. This later turned into a fullblown addiction, as it would temporarily relieve all of my symptoms and make me feel what I imagined was "normal." At first, the alcohol did for me what antidepressants never did. When I drank, there were no fight or flight feelings, there was no sadness or hurt, there were no panic attacks or anxiety, and I began to feel like my childhood self again. I was temporarily free from all the baggage. I eventually became physically dependent on alcohol and drinking experiences gradually became more negative. It eventually got to the point where I'd rarely have positive drinking experiences and I'd blackout fairly easily.

Drinking was a hard thing to come to terms with for me. It seemed like my peers in their early to midtwenties were drinking heavily, without issues. It wasn't until my blackout episodes led me into legal problems and losing relationships, that I began to take notice. I became more depressed than I had ever been before and the alcohol had stopped helping my symptoms. Eventually, the drinking made my symptoms worse.

I began drinking just to not feel withdrawal symptoms. The withdrawal was the most uncomfortable physical sensation that I have ever experienced. I constantly had a horrible sensation with my nerves in my fingers and teeth. My PTSD and anxiety-related symptoms were out of control. It seemed like I was constantly in a state of fight-or-flight and I lost an unhealthy amount of weight from not being able to hold down solid food anymore.

Over the next few years, I kept fighting alcohol addiction. I came to realize just how interrelated the drinking was to my depression. For anyone who has ever been depressed, it's very easy to lose motivation and give up on long-term goals, especially when stressful events occur. I had a series of events spiral me back into depression and eventually drinking after periods of sobriety. During this period of intermittent sobriety, I lost two friends to their addictions, and I was also facing legal issues from a DUI and a series of false allegations from a disgruntled ex-friend. Despite these stressors, I somehow managed to make it through two master's degrees and three years of doctoral school, all while working. Although this time period had some major accomplishments, it added to the intense levels of stress that I was already facing.

Looking back at this volatile period of change, some of the best and worst events occurred in my entire life. My professional life took off in many ways, but my social life suffered. My drinking took a toll on my relationship with my family as well. It was my will to live that eventually set me on the right path. I began doing dangerous things while drinking that could have killed me or (even worse) someone else. I realized that for as awful as I felt and as unhappy as I was, I no longer wanted to die. I had spent so much time as a youth thinking about suicide, that I forgot what it was like to have long-term dreams. After a few close calls with death, I realized that not only did I not want to die, but I actually wanted to live and be happy.

This was really when things started to get better. Although I've relapsed and have taken steps backward since the beginning of this journey, this realization kept me fighting to progress. Today, my life is very positive and full of continual growth as a person. Professionally, I ran my own business over the past few years and have enjoyed volunteering in leadership roles for several local non-profits. Personally, I now have the best group of friends I've ever had and I am closer than ever with my family.

However, I'd be lying if I said that things were perfect and that I'm cured of anything. I've had slips with my drinking, there are moments where I really want to drink, and I still have days where my depression kicks my butt. However, these are less frequent occurrences, I'm better at both preventing and ending lapses when they do occur, and I've celebrated some of the longest periods of sobriety and happiest moments of my life over the past few years. I also have built a strong support network through communities I've joined and healthier friendships. A hard part of getting better, for me, was cutting out people that I cared about but who were toxic for my recovery and growth.

Mental health maintenance is often a life-long journey. I currently do not go to therapy of any kind, but there may be a time where I will need some support again. I take low doses of Prozac and Naltrexone (an alcohol/opioid anti-craving drug), but I may need higher doses later on and / or additional medications. I think it's easy to view relapses with substances or going back to therapy as regressing, but this couldn't be further from the truth. I am not the same person as I was when I started this journey and I can only keep working to make myself the happiest and healthiest that I can possibly be. For every one step that I take backward, I try and take three steps forward. Sometimes I still mess up, but it just encourages me to make up for it in positive ways.

I believe that helping other people has been vital to progress. When I was at my worst moments, I can recall being entirely focused on my own issues and tuning everyone else out. When I forced myself to overcome how I'm feeling to help others or open up to others, it makes a world of a difference. It's healthy to remember that there are things bigger than ourselves.

Realizing that there is a larger picture also can create a solid sense of meaning and belonging. Modern behavioral treatment models are helpful, but can often overlook existential issues and how they contribute to

127

mental health. What gets you up in the morning? What is your meaning or purpose? What do you want out of life? What is happiness and success to you? While the answers to these questions may change over time, I do believe thinking about them and having a general idea is important to feeling healthy.

The narrative that we tell ourselves can help us function or cause great dysfunction. It has also helped me to not identify myself by my depression, traumatic experiences, or addiction. I believe calling someone "mentally ill," "depressed," an "alcoholic," or any other definitive term related to mental health is counterproductive. As therapists, we are trained to use phrases like "a person with depression." Phrasing disorders this way detaches identify from the disorder. It conveys the message that there is much more to a person than their adversity. A disorder is just one part of an individual and should be communicated as such. This is also why I think developing hobbies, networks, and habits outside of support groups can be just as helpful as therapy. Developing things that have nothing to do with a dilemma can help an individual get outside of that dilemma. These are just a few things that have helped me over the years and that I continue to practice and develop to this day.

The moment that we stop growing is the moment that we start dying. Some research indicates that people tend to avoid discomfort more than they seek pleasure. This can make motivation extremely difficult when the path to mental wellness is full of short-term discomfort and delayed outcomes. It is easier to just keep avoiding therapy, continue drinking to cope or blame everyone else for the negative outcomes of behavior. However, the easier road often leads to negative results.

It's when we break down, get mad, feel hopeless, get motivated, yet decide to live that true change can occur. It's a long road, it's not an easy road, but I don't believe anyone ever reaches a place where life is constantly an easy ride. However, it does get better, there is hope, and we can find contentment in every moment. Being grounded in the present is a tall order, as the past and future always seem to be lurking nearby. Yet, it is now and today that change can start and with each day, we can feel just a little bit more alive.

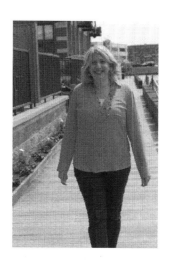

Carrie Reichartz

Carrie Reichartz, Executive Director for the I Am Enough In Christ Women's Conferences, as well as founder and Executive Director of Infinitely More takes frequent mission trips to Kenya to work with people affected by trauma and pregnancy issues. She has a true passion for children and helping people travel through trauma into triumph by inspiring them through her personal story. You can contact her and find more about her work at InfinitelyMoreLife.org, IAmEnoughInChrist.com, and the Kenya mission work at MercysLight.org.

My Journey of Turning Trauma to Triumph: From Childhood Sexual Abuse into an Amazing Life

By Carrie Reichartz

"... Since God assured us, "I'll never let you down, never walk off and leave you," we can boldly quote, God is there, ready to help; I'm fearless no matter what. Who or what can get to me?

– Hebrews 13:5-6 The Message (MSG)

Do you need hope for the future amid struggles with mental health? I hope my story will bring you that.

My story of mental health is unique as is everyone's. For me, I do not know life before sexual abuse. It started for me, at the hand of an extended family member, long before my first memory. I only know this because it presents itself in my life through smells, words, and other triggers.

Later in life, I had two other sexual assault situations and many other life dramas and traumas. I bounced back by putting "controls" over my life in place. Putting these in place let my mind believe I had control over life and the situations. These traumas and the resulting "controls" I put in my life left me feeling abandoned, alone, and afraid. My life was full of extreme fear - terror; extreme shyness–silence; and being completely emotionally shut down.

At the lowest point in my life–my body had betrayed me — that left me with no choice than to admit I didn't have control over things. After many years of healing, my life now couldn't be better. That is what I want for you as well. Join me through my journey of turning trauma into triumph.

Life During Mental Health Challenges

The trauma of sexual abuse and assaults left me living in extreme fear. It was more like terror. Everything felt out of my control and even my influence. So I created rituals in my life that gave me the feeling of control and safety.

I needed to stay one step ahead of everyone and then I could keep everything under control. Failure to prepare would ensure something bad would happen.

So, I just needed to think two or three steps ahead of everyone and everything else. If I did this, then I would be safe. This kept my mind racing at all times to ensure I was ahead of the game and didn't miss anything.

For example, never having my back to a door in a room would help me make sure I knew everything going on around me. Going to sleep wearing a full set of clothes was another example. If I just did something to prevent the assaults – they would never happen again. I just needed to be extra diligent, vigilant, and careful. My wearing of the "right" clothing would prevent future attacks and keep me in control of my life.

These types of behaviors gave me the illusion of control and safety in my life which brought muchneeded peace and comfort to my mind. But I felt alone and afraid, and my mind was on constant anxious alert.

The extreme trauma also led me inward so I was extremely shy. I was shy to the point of remaining silent. My mom once told me that my kindergarten teacher was going to call social services because I was so quiet.

I would not even open up and share with my nuclear family. My mom signed me up for gymnastics. After the first year or two, I hated it. I didn't want to go nor did I enjoy it. I didn't share that with my mom for over ten years. I tried to be invisible. If I didn't exist, no one could see me and no future bad things would occur. The shyness resulting from the sexual abuse left me feeling alone and afraid.

Also, the extreme trauma had completely cut me off and shut me down emotionally. Imagine turning your feelings off at the age of two or three years old? How would you function in life when situations arose? After the second round of sexual assaults in my pre-teens, I knew I was forever changed. I could literally feel the little bit of current life that I did have fall away from me. It was as if the broken shards of glass that were held so loosely together after the sexual abuse were now totally shattered into tiny pieces that could never be put back together.

I remember a moment in the bathroom, feeling that shattered self for a moment and then turning it all off. It was too much for me to process. Too much for me to handle.

I turned off my feelings and replaced them with control.

I turned off my mind to try to not hurt anymore. In fact, for many years after that day in the bathroom, I didn't remember what had happened; I had turned it off so tightly. I lived for years without the memory coming to mind.

For many years, life went on as normal to everyone around me. I went to school. I didn't draw attention to myself. I didn't act up. I did what I needed to do to stay under the radar–I got good enough grades and did what everyone told me to do. All of this facade kept me feeling abandoned, alone, and afraid, but it was all I knew.

FLOODGATES OPEN

Out of nowhere, it all came flooding back … several years later, while watching an after-school special on TV as I was working on my homework in my room. The theme of the show was date rape. In a few scenes, a girl was yelling "STOP" over and over again. At that exact moment, all the memories came flooding back of the abuse and the feelings of being shattered in the bathroom that day.

I didn't know what to do. Not one person came to mind to reach out to for help. I couldn't trust anyone. They were all possibly going to hurt me and I would let my guard down. What if they didn't believe me? Why would they believe me, this happened years ago? And worse, what if I shared what I went through and then no one did anything? That would hurt even more than the current pain. So, to be stoic, I just held it in. I just kept chugging along in the facade of life being fine. All the while, it led me deeper into the need to control and feelings of being abandoned,

135

alone, and afraid.

There was a moment of possible hope in my late teens where I reached out in desperation to my best friend for help. We were at a party. Someone there looked exactly like the person that had raped me. I begged my friend to leave the party with me. She refused. After some drama, I shared with her what happened to me and why I wanted to leave. To summarize a very tearful and difficult emotional situation, I left the party alone. I was abandoned, alone, and afraid again; now caused by the first person I had reached out to for help, who I thought cared about me.

This failed attempt to reach out for help clearly confirmed my feelings of being abandoned, alone, and afraid. I was abandoned, alone and afraid and no one would change that.

After that moment I locked the doors of my heart. I didn't think about this situation. I didn't mention it. I didn't have any reason to. I moved forward telling myself that the situations were in the past and they were not affecting me. I didn't know it, but I was locking myself further into abandoned, alone and afraid feelings.

All this controlling, covering, masking, and hiding moved me into depression and deep anxiety. Life started to spiral downward. Drinking, partying, and dating boys (or men) that were not good for me financially, emotionally, or physically, seemed the only way to live. I got involved in an extremely abusive dating relationship which resulted in very difficult situations.

From that low point of my life, I changed direction. I moved from what appeared as a downward spiral to what appeared to be coming back up. I switched to achievement. If I knew enough I could keep myself safe so I want on to law school. I worked three jobs and went to school part-time. I got married because that was the next right step. I had kids. On the outside, things looked perfect. But on the inside, my first husband struggled with alcohol and drug abuse, pushing my need to control him, the kids, and myself even more.

I thought if I accomplished enough, I could save my husband and everyone would love and accept me and I would not be abandoned, alone and afraid anymore. I thought I would be accepted, loved, and safe. This achievement strategy increased anxiety in me. I needed to control a lot of things, especially situations beyond my control, to ensure that I was loved, accepted and safe.

A Pivotal Point in the Downfall

I did a great job of keeping up the illusion of control, at

least from the outside, until ...

I had a major health crisis. I had a PE (pulmonary embolism, a blood clot that went from my leg to my lung). PE's are usually fatal. During my eight-day hospital stay, a news reporter in Iraq died of a PE as he exited a tanker he had been moving in. The news kept playing it over and over and over and over.

Listening to this news coverage left me with mantras in my own head "you should be dead. This should have killed you. It will kill you. You are not safe." Words and feelings I had heard earlier in life from the perpetrators of sexual abuse and assault.

My whole life I have felt abandoned, alone, and afraid. I had finally found a strategy of achievement to pull me out of that pit. And now, I never felt more abandoned, alone, and afraid. I was now afraid of my own body. I had always been afraid of others around me, but now it was inside me. My own body was betraying me.

I had spent so many years doing what I thought was a great job controlling every situation in my life - alcoholic husband, kids, work, school, life. Now, I had no idea how to even start to take control of this. Then, one week after I got out of the hospital, still unable to walk or work, my husband left me and the kids (they were only five and three years old at the time) to be with a former friend of mine who he had been seeing for several months before that.

Pivotal Point in Healing: Admitting to Another

Not able to deal with life situations psychologically, I made an appointment with a psychologist to deal with the health and marital issues. I had to answer many questions as she completed my intake. One or two of the questions asked about sexual abuse and assault. I left those blank. I considered lying and just checking the NO box. But instead, for some reason, I left them blank.

Long story short, after a session or two I unlocked that door of my heart and talked about the sexual abuse and rape situations I had experienced, all the while assuring the psychologist that these situations had no bearing on my current life situation. I didn't think about those things ever. They were not affecting me at all.

As we moved through individual and group counseling, things were moving nicely. I was finding healing and wholeness in the mists of struggles. Letting go of my need to control, just a little bit. My psychologist recommended a course and experience at a place called the Center for Creative Learning in Milwaukee, Wisconsin. This is where I finally started fully processing and owning my feelings for the first time in my life. Tears were flowing and toxins were leaving my body!

I had never felt so happy or free in all my life. Life was amazing, most of the time. If I watched the right *Oprah* show, read the right book, took the right class, attended the right workshop, then life was great and perfect. If I didn't, then life would revert back to old ways of feeling and thinking. It really turned into another thing to control. At least it offered great results, but I was still trying to control my life.

A few years after this, a friend I met through the Center asked me to join her in going to church. I told her I wasn't interested. I had grown up in the church and it didn't have anything to offer me. She was persistent. After hours and hours of persuading me, I finally caved in and told myself – it is one hour; just do it to shut her up.

It was a trip that would change my life forever. I can't share all of the details here for there is no end to the change this has made in my life. I finally found a "person" that I could fully trust to help me through ALL my life struggles, big and small. Finally, Someone to pull me out from under the paralyzing fear, crippling shyness, and emotional numbness.

Though I even hate to write it, because it feels so cliché, but it is true. My life has been absolutely transformed in every area, in every way. Now, this is not about church, the building. It is about a relationship - a relationship with Jesus, not a list of rules, which is what I thought it was when I was growing up. I know a place to find my answers now– not the next right book, *Oprah* show, movie, workshop, etc. not that all of those cannot be of help – the final and true answers I will find for my life are in the Bible. I would love to share more and more on this, so feel free to reach out to me!

Life Now

My life after working on healing and finding a relationship with Jesus is AMAZING! I actually, at times, feel a tiny bit of gratitude for the tough experiences because, without those tough experiences, I wouldn't be able to handle all that I am doing now.

I have been able to inspire others to turn their traumas into triumphs. Through personal friendships with those around me, I am able to relate to people's pain and be one example of pain being a pit-stop on the way to something better, giving them hope and inspiration.

In larger settings, I work with a small crew of people to show hope and inspiration via conferences we produce in the United States through *Infinitely More*, a non-profit I founded during my healing journey. Writing books and small-group coaching are also ways this

141

experience is helping people in the U.S. turn their trauma into triumph.

However, the thing I am most awestruck about through this healing journey is a project in Mombasa, Kenya called Mercy's Light Family. I never wanted to travel the world. I was hoping to hit the 50 states someday – minus Alaska and Hawaii because they were too far.

But one day in 2008, God brought me on a journey to Mombasa, Kenya, and my life has never been the same. You can read about that whole journey in *From Lawyer to Missionary: A Journey to Kenya and Back Again.*

It ties into our journey together here, starting in 2012. That's when I, with the help of God and many volunteers, started working on founding a pregnancy crisis and trauma center for a rural village near Mombasa, Kenya. It is a maternity home for girls who are pregnant specifically because of sexual trauma.

In 2018, the doors opened and we currently have four girls and their four babies in our center working on healing through love, trauma counseling, and Biblical Counseling. These are girls who would otherwise be left in the streets to die. Because of feeling the same feelings of being abandoned, alone and afraid, they would abort or abandon their babies. Instead, because of my journey, we have been able to provide help and healing to these girls and life to their babies! You can see more about what we do with the girls and babies at our center at MercysLight.org.

A Word Of Advice

To anyone struggling, I would say– you are not alone. Don't let anyone convince you that you are. Don't convince yourself that you are. Get help from a professional and let them help you move forward in your life. People want to help you. Reach out.

I would follow that up to say, don't stay stuck in the psychologists' chair either. We need someone to help us work through the trauma for sure. Do not do that alone. Also, don't sit on that couch for years and years and years. Use that couch as a safe place to land and process what has happened to you. Then use that as the start of a new life and living. Use it to start dreaming again.

These events don't need to define you or keep you down. Let them be the events that raise you high above and fly you to help the person next to you. If you are struggling in this area – feeling stuck with the counselor – life coaching can be a place to find that footing again. At Infinitely More Life – Dream, Learn and Fly, that is exactly what we help people do!

I pray that for you – a life full of hope!

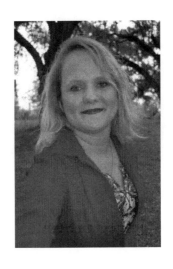

Dana Lambert-Hodge

Dana Lambert-Hodge is a South Carolina native, currently living in the Blue Ridge Mountains. She lives with her loving husband, Donald and her four children, Winston, Emmalee, Laycie, and Jackson. She enjoys reading, writing, photography, blogging on her personal website at *Luv'N Lambert Life* and speaking out about the things that mean the most to her. She often shares her struggles of living with epilepsy, depression, and the joys of homeschooling her children on her website. She finds solace in nature, sitting by the flowing rivers in the mountains that surround her every day.

Facebook Page:

https://www.facebook.com/luvnlambertlife

Blog: http://www.luvnlambertlife.com

Finding My Own Happiness While Living With Depression

By Dana Lambert-Hodge

Promise me you'll always remember: You're braver than you believe, and stronger than you seem, and smarter than you think.

– Christopher Robin

All of my life, I have been surrounded by those who suffer from different levels of mental health challenges. Even as a child, I was affected in some way. My parents and my grandparents have battled with their own mental health challenges throughout their lives which, of course, has trickled down into mine.

I was born to a mother who has had manic depression as long as I can remember, a father who was never around me, and a stepfather who was mentally controlling and abusive for most of my life. My mother was born to a father who had schizophrenia with multiple personality disorder, and a

147

mother whose depression developed after unexpectedly losing a child, which she kept hidden for most of her own life. This affected my mother's mental health deeply.

My mental health challenges began as a child with mild issues of depression. When I was six, I had a deep sadness when my 16-year-old brother left home because of the abuse he endured from my stepfather. I felt a deep sadness again when my older sister left home after high school many years later. I felt abandoned by their leaving. I was hurt by the sadness in my mother's eyes as her children left her as well.

As a child, I didn't understand their reasons and having a depressed mother did not help me cope with the changes. I began to harden my feelings even at a young age, often feeling like I needed to make up for them, or simply doing everything I could so they would not be there. When my stepfather would start arguments with my mother, I would often try to intervene. I would stand up to him and take his abuse. This was just life for us and in some ways, I guess I probably felt it was love. I would protect my mother from his verbal attacks in an effort to combat her sadness and pain.

I didn't understand then just how deep her depression ran. Even for her to seek help for her depression was a huge battle with him. He saw therapy as a useless waste and would tell her repeatedly nothing was wrong with her. He shamed her need for seeking help. I also did not understand why my biological father was never around. The times he would come by were infrequent and my memories of him are vague and few. When I was 13, he called to say that he was dying, but I was on the phone with my friend, and like a typical teenager, I just wanted to return to my call. It was the last time I would talk with him, as he died shortly after. I never had a real relationship with his family after his death, nor before, to be honest.

Around this same time, my best friend attempted suicide through overdosing. Even as a girl, she was unhappy with life and struggled to deal with her depression. Her attempt was unsuccessful but I will never forget visiting her in the hospital and seeing her face stained with the charcoal that had been used to induce vomiting and save her life.

At 17, I met my first husband through mutual friends. He seemed wonderful, but he had his hidden secrets. He was seven years older than me and I was inexperienced in life. I didn't realize how little he had his life together because, at the time, I knew very little about life myself. We dated for two years and then we got married. A year later we had our son, and then 26 months afterward, our daughter. We struggled financially. He wanted me home with the kids, so I didn't work outside the home and he wasn't the best provider. There were many times when bills did not get paid and the lights would get shut off, or the gas would run out. There were many days when landlords would pound on our door wanting their rent money.

On top of this, he had a serious addiction to porn and women. He gave our bill money to the girls he would visit, mostly strippers I think. He became involved with drugs and his temper was negatively affected by this lifestyle. One night in anger, he lifted me by my throat and tossed me across the bed. This was the final straw for me. It was not the life I wanted for myself or for my children, so I left him.

This relationship was followed by another - more abuse and more struggles. I gave birth to my second daughter. This person made me feel so lost. I was at fault for everything, for all the issues in my relationships, for the abuse, for their anger. I was at fault for bills and whatever else was wrong. I now realize that he was a lot like my stepfather. The relationship ended as well and the time period that followed was extremely difficult for both my children and me.

Another relationship came, and I thought it was everything I wanted: love, happiness, a home for myself and my kids. But it didn't take long to realize I was where I was not wanted. I spent six years there battling ghosts I could not defeat. I seem to attract narcissists. This particular man had Post Traumatic Syndrome Disorder (PTSD) from an accident he had been in years prior and he also had a serious addiction to sex, porn and a deep infatuation with women. I felt it was different from my first husband, however, and I really thought it was love. I am ashamed to say, it never was. I stayed because I didn't want to admit I had failed once again and I didn't want my children to lose another home.

When I became pregnant with my son, he seemed to grow worse. He claimed I forced him into having this child. He claimed I tied him down in a relationship that he never wanted. He told me over and over again that he did not want my son. When I almost miscarried him, his father had to tell him to go to the ER to check on us. Even when he was born, he seemed unphased by his birth.

In the end, his family became the abusers, siding with him because in their eyes he could do no wrong. I was the bad girl in this situation, doing him wrong while he cheated on me every chance he got. Their excuse was that we were not married, so I did not matter.

After one argument we had, he left and went to his parents. His father came over to scream at me, saying that I needed to leave, furthering the abuse and trauma from him and his family. He felt because it was his land, that he had the right to react in this way. He never asked why we argued or who was at fault because the fault was never on my ex, his child.

It took him flaunting his relationships in front of me, shoving me with his entire weight across my kitchen, throwing me into the washer and dryer in our laundry room, moving it several inches from the force of the attack, for me to realize enough was enough. After this, I would leave the house and stay with friends because he did not want me there. Then he and his family would use that against me, claiming I was cheating on him when he was the one cheating the entire time.

I reached out for help with the local center for abused women because I had nowhere to go and no idea what to do next. When my ex and his family found out, they made life even worse for me. They filed for eviction to remove me and my children from our home of six years.

During this time, my mother had also been living in a home on their property. They filed to evict her as well. I received calls from her telling me I was causing her to lose her home when really it was my ex's passions and his family forcing all of these things to happen. This sent her spiraling into a manic episode which led to further problems for me. Out of her own fear, she made untrue accusations and statements to those around her, causing them to reach out to authorities to attempt to "help." I had to correct these issues created by people who unknowingly had fallen into her paranoia to keep from having more issues as we moved.

Throughout my life, I have had to deal with my mother's mental health challenges. Before my first marriage ended, my stepfather, the man who had raised me, passed away. My mother went into a deep depression and I was unable to help. I sent her to my siblings so they could help, but she has not been the same since. She lost a great deal with his death: her home, cars, and stability. 14 years later, she still has not regained these things or seemingly any hope with her life.

A mother with a mental illness weighs heavily. Somehow over the years, she's always ended up back with me. My siblings have a hard time handling her ups and downs, and do not seem to understand her mental health challenges. Her mood swings and her deep emotions are often too much for them to handle. They leave that to me to deal with daily and mostly alone.

At the end of my last relationship, when the world around me was falling apart and I had no idea what to do next, I began therapy. I knew from my mother's life that it was important to take care of myself. I was diagnosed with mild depression, caused by my circumstances. Truthfully, I really wanted it all to an end: my life, the pain, the lies and cheating, the hurt my mother had caused over the years. I just wanted life to be over. I was 35 and had no idea what I was

153

going to do, where I was going to go, and I was tired of trying to find love and happiness only to fail. Nothing I did was good enough.

At my darkest, I sat in my car in a Walmart parking lot contemplating how to end my life. I convinced myself that my children would be better off without me. No one loved me: not my ex nor my mother, friends were fake and life was not worth it. My entire world was nothing but chaos. I had no home, nowhere to go, no money because I had not worked in years because of my children's battles with epilepsy and other health issues. There was no one for me to turn to.

When I had reached out to the abuse center, I was told they had no housing and if we went into their shelter, I had to put my children, who had been homeschooled from birth, into a public school. I realized this was discrimination but at the time I was stuck. It only helped to increase my depression. In the end, we did not go there for housing because after all we'd been through, I was not going to be forced to compromise our lifestyle and values. It's the one thing I stood firm on for our family. I wanted to keep my children's lives as normal as I was able to.

I continued seeing my therapist. She was an amazing source of strength and guidance for me. She supported my decisions as I moved forward. She encouraged me to keep going and helped me feel I could find a way out of my situation. She promised me there would be better times ahead and that I just had to get past these hurdles to find them. Even though at that moment, I could only see the darkness and feel immense sadness, she was a shining light helping me through.

We did finally find a home and move. We began again in a new town. We started over.

I met my now-husband at this time and he helped me to accomplish all of these things as a friend. He wasn't perfect and he had his own challenges along the way. Our beginning was not an easy one because of my broken heart and his own personal issues, but we have overcome them altogether. He too has depression, but we support each other on our path and walk through things with each other to get past it all. We lift each other up, hold each other when necessary and push each other to do better every day.

My husband has helped me heal. He also helped me see my worth. He values me like no one ever has. He loves me unconditionally despite my past and my present flaws. He came into my life when I needed him the most and he has taught me love and compassion. He stands beside me through all of the challenges we face. He is there for my children every day as well, loving them as much as I do.

My children have also kept me going through all of

this. They needed me and they still do. Their love and their precious smiles healed my heart and lift my depression even today. I had to continue to be strong for them. I had to be more for them. I had to keep going because they needed me. My presence is important in their lives and theirs in mine. They make my life worth living every day.

When we moved, I also found a new therapist who helped me see my worth. He was a great blessing to me, encouraging me to develop my interests and find happiness in myself. He helped me learn how to forgive my mother, though forgiveness will always be a work in progress for me. He encouraged me to journal and get my feelings out instead of keeping them boxed up, leading me to write. He also helped me to see I have PTSD and anxiety, along with my depression, and helped me learn coping skills to deal with these issues.

All of these people offered me the support and love I needed to help me keep moving forward. They helped me to see myself. They helped me to build a stronger me. They gathered me up and helped me to see my value and purpose. They showed me I deserve love, despite the voices of my past. They showed me that I deserve to live a full and happy life.

Support has been a big help too in moving forward with my life. The support of my kids, my husband, and my friends have helped me to get through so much.

They allow me to vent, cry and even to scream if I need to. I'm thankful that I have a great support system.

I am still dealing with my mother's mental health, but I have coping techniques to get me through. It's been a long road of forgiveness and some days it's still hard for me because of all she's done to me and my children in the past. I know the disease she has is not her, but daily affects how she thinks, feels and reacts to things. Because of that, I can forgive her.

I am now proactive in speaking out about my mother's mental health before she can tell mistruths which may later cause our family issues. This doesn't always go over favorably with people who do not understand our life together, but most people are sympathetic and understanding overall. The ones who don't understand though, weigh heavily on me and it's those times I feel my depression sneaking in on me. I worry, but I just keep myself going and I remind myself that I am doing what is best in order to protect my family first.

For me, my PTSD is the hardest to deal with. It's triggered by these past issues with my mother, from the abuse I have endured in my life both with my parents and my exes and also from my children's battles with epilepsy over the years. I have nightmares about my children not waking up after a seizure. I worry constantly we will miss a seizure and

157

it will cause permanent issues or worse, death for my children. I become fearful if I'm away from my children for too long, even if I'm just at the store. I worry about my mother saying the wrong thing from one of her manic episodes and what repercussions that might cause. I get anxiety when I'm in crowded places or intense traffic keeping me from getting home to my kids quickly when I am away for appointments or grocery shopping.

I get anxiety over many other things as well.

At my recent doctor's appointment, my physician stated I have too much stress. She said I do not sleep enough. She is right! I get little sleep and I almost never rest when I do sleep. Stress comes from managing my household. There is no one who can pick up the slack. I'm the mediator between everyone and everything involving my home falls on my shoulders. This is what often happens in a blended family.

This doesn't get me down, though. I feel no sadness like I used to. I am tired, but I know when I need to shut my door and shut everything out. I find that sitting on my front porch in the fresh air and sunshine helps greatly. Talking with friends is also a great release and simply spending time with my husband and my children is the best encouragement of all.

My biggest challenge is still my mother's depression.

We are working on a better health plan for her, which I hope will help her become more of the mother that my siblings and I used to have. That will take time and it is a process, but I am hopeful for her. I cherish the years we have left together despite our past, and I cherish the time she has left with my siblings and her grandchildren as well. Life is all too short.

I still journal. I write on my blog, I share online and I write privately as well. I enjoy looking back at where I have been and how far I have come. It no longer makes me sad, but I see joy in my future. Journaling and writing help me to get my feelings out while helping me to keep the sadness from building up inside of me. It releases emotions I may otherwise hold inside. I can honestly say that it's been a long time since I felt truly sad at all.

I have also become a calmer person, especially with my children. I removed many toxic people from my life and that has helped a great deal. I blocked them online as well, so they don't upset me, and I don't see them or have to deal with them. I avoid them in public when necessary. I have no patience for drama, so I stop it before it can start, and I am learning to walk away even though it's hard sometimes.

I have also become a better parent. I feel more in control now, though some days are still slightly overwhelming. I see my own worth. I see my children's worth as well. I want to see all their dreams come true and stand beside them as they walk through their life's paths. I want to be the mother they want and need me to be.

I yell less and I try to speak to their hearts more. I show love to them more often than I used to. I no longer use harsh punishment as I did when I was a young mother, but I listen and I cuddle and reach out to their hearts instead. I am working on breaking the cycle that my own parents created in me by learning a better way and showing that to my children instead.

Love is the way to go, and love can overcome all.

I lead my children to see the good in others. I've shown forgiveness to their grandmother which they have seen, and I have encouraged them to show her the same forgiveness as well. We do not build hate in our home. I encourage my children to find beauty in every day and to look for hope in the darkness. I encourage them to show kindness to strangers and to embrace friends.

I now speak out for all the things I have been through in my life. I share about our epilepsy, about mental illness, about the abuse I have endured and about the daily challenges we have lived through and are still battling each day. I try to show others that they are not alone in these battles. I try to encourage others to speak out as well and share their own stories. Our testimonies speak life every day.

I am teaching myself and my children to create our own happiness. I am trying to show them that happiness resides within each of us, that our passions, our thoughts, our feelings, and our emotions all mean something and all matter. I'm even trying to show my mother that love outweighs all and that life is so much more than depression filled unhappiness. I strive to see the beauty of tomorrow over the darkness of the past days.

I am not my challenges or my past. My children and I are not my mother, nor the mental illness we have. There is an alternative way. We do not have to continue the cycles of yesterday. Changing life and creating an environment filled with love, finding joy and allowing happiness in our lives can change your world.

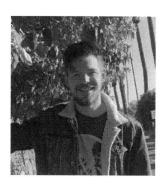

Karsten Penkacik

Born in Illinois, Karsten Penkacik is the oldest of 12 siblings and is currently pursuing a Bachelor's in Criminal Justice in Arizona. He works full time while attending school. He is currently employed by a beer distribution. His career goal is to become a lawyer working in criminal felony cases. Karsten can be reached at kpenkacik@gmail.com.

Why Knowing Your Worth Is Important

By Karsten Penkacik

"Everything happens for a reason"

Over the past couple of years, I've realized how important a person's mental health is, especially when it comes to forming and maintaining relationships, whether romantic, familial or friendships. Maintaining my mental health wasn't something I really thought about growing up; life just seemed so much simpler than it actually is. There were fewer worries, less stress, and less self-doubt. Life wasn't perfect, but it seemed to only carry a normal amount of worry and stress. The mental challenges I faced weren't always there. For the most part, I think I had a happy childhood.

I had to grow up sooner than most, but it didn't seem to impact the way I acted around others, aside from the intense shyness I had when I was a kid. It wasn't until my teenage years that I began to notice a shift in what I deemed a normal level of mental pressure. One instance that I remember was when I was talking to my friend's mom about a girl that I had started

163

dating. She had given me a ride home, and the subject had come up in conversation. I don't remember the exact words spoken, but what I do remember is how she said that I would never be good enough and to date someone in my league. That hit me hard coming from someone that I respected.

Saying that I wouldn't be enough for someone just drove its way into my heart and lodged itself there, gnawing away at my self-confidence. The words echoed through my mind for a few months after the fact, and unfortunately, it wouldn't be the last time that someone I respected would say something similar to me. The whole experience messed me up deeper than I thought and that's when my self-image and level of worth started degrading.

I can't emphasize how important it is to know your self-worth and to know just how important you actually are. It may not always seem like it, but you are worth so much more than you realize. It took me a long time to realize that, and I'm still working every day to remind myself of how much I matter to everyone around me. Not knowing your worth can ruin you from the inside out.

One of the darkest times in my life came during my first year of college. I had decided to live in the dorms before finding out that my whole family was moving out of state, and since I was going to school, I stayed behind. I was making a life here, so I wasn't too upset about my family moving on to another place, but after a while, I began to feel alone. On top of that, I was still trying to figure out what I wanted to do with my life, and I felt like I was figuring that out much later than I should have.

Everything hit me at once, and it felt so overwhelming. I felt like I was drowning and couldn't swim up fast enough. I began to feel like an adult, and I started to long for the days when I was surrounded by friends and didn't feel like every decision I made was a bad one. With all of my friends and family so far away from me, my descent into depression worsened, and the people I was taking advice from didn't help the matter either.

To calm myself down I would take walks late at night, mostly around midnight to the parking garage offcampus. It helped to have a quiet space away from everything. I would take that time to talk to God and try to get mad at Him for everything I was dealing with. However, I couldn't because I felt like everything that I was dealing with was my fault.

I had a few days where I felt completely hopeless like I no longer had any control over my life, and that the downward spiral would just continue. I will not lie, I would just look over the railing of the top level of that parking garage from time to time and think about if my problems were worth me jumping over the edge. They never were, I held onto hope that things would get better, and that's what got me through that season.

My depression took a while to improve and even reached a point where I never wanted to get out of bed. Eventually, I left that school for the semester and decided to not return the following school year. Sometimes you have to get yourself out of an environment that brings out the worst in you so you can work to get better. It's not always as easy as just deciding that you're not returning, but it's worth the effort for the betterment of your mental health.

In terms of a romantic relationship, it's much more difficult as I'm finding out. You have to accept that someone can see you in a way that you cannot see yourself, and it's even more difficult to understand why they would feel that way about you. From my experience, it made it hard for me to enjoy the relationship I was in due to the worry of whether they would still feel the same way about me once they got to know me more. I felt like I wasn't anything special, and that there were far better guys out there than me. That mindset led me to make rash decisions and ones that affected not only me but others as well.

I wish I knew then what I know now, and that those decisions could have been avoided. I like to believe that everything happens for a reason, and that led me to seek help with everything that I was facing and to make a better effort in managing it. It was hard for me to ask for help, but doing this on my own wasn't working. I could see how the things I was dealing with were affecting those around me and the people that got close to me. The change didn't happen overnight, and it took quite a bit of effort on my part to get where I am now.

The hardest part for me was learning to enjoy life again. I couldn't remember how I used to enjoy the simple things, and where it started, so I didn't know how to get back there. But thankfully I had someone that I could talk to, and who could point me in the right direction. Currently, I'm working every day to keep myself from slipping back into my depressive state, and finding new ways to enjoy the little things in life, by making time for myself and doing the things I love. It's always good to have a plan in place for when you start to feel yourself slipping. You're going to have challenging days, but keep your head up high, and know that you're going to get through it.

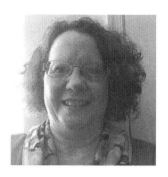

Carol Strang

Carol Strang is a wife, mother and education assistant who resides in New Jersey. Carol has been ministering to women since 2016 and shares her testimony of self-discovery and healing from her long battle with insecurity. Her purpose and passion are for women to know their true identity in Christ, and be free from condemnation. Carol is an inspirational author, blogger, and speaker. She is devoted to the Lord and runs her own women's podcast. Find out more at https://carolatvictoriouslivinghome.blog

Don't Let People's Opinions Dictate Your Life!

By Carol Strang

"There are two lasting bequests we can give our children. One is roots. The other is wings."

– Hodding Carter, Jr.

My first unpleasant authoritative incident occurred in my kindergarten class. My teacher told me in a forceful tone that I "should color in the lines." Our Catholic school comprised primarily strict nuns who had mean personalities. On one occasion, I was summoned to the Mother Superior's office and received several slaps on my knuckles, because I wasn't supposed to play tag around the buses. However, my accomplice escaped! Another time I received a written punishment from a teacher because I smiled in class! This was not a good environment for me. I received low grades and my confidence lessened.

In my neighborhood, I had three "so-called" friends. I would play Barbies, hopscotch, roller skate, and other childhood games. One time, the girls had a Barbie clothes exchange. Well, they went home with my mom's beautiful hand-made clothes, and I was stuck with ugly Barbie outfits. One girl destroyed my lifesaver doll and then denied it. These girls would ridicule me, pick fights, and shout accusations that weren't true. I even had to quit Brownies (a Girl Scout program) because of their unkind behavior.

When I entered the fourth grade, my parents moved to South Jersey and enrolled me in public school. My grades steadily improved and my confidence went up. The following year, I entered fifth grade, and happily sang in the choir. Sadly, in sixth grade, my dad stopped taking me to choir practice.

Sixth grade was my best year academically and socially. I achieved excellent grades, my classmates respected me, and I was the teacher's pet. I adored my social studies and math teacher - he made learning fun! I even had a handsome boyfriend for a brief period, but we had to break-up because my parents wouldn't allow me to date. This was the one year that I developed lots of plans and dreams.

Unfortunately, seventh grade was my worst year. A new pretty girl was making my life miserable. She would make fun of me and my wardrobe. She turned all my friends against me.

There was also another girl who made fun of me. She was African-American and the other girl was

Caucasian. She would verbally abuse me and pick fights and tried to take money from me. This all started because I accidentally hit her with my locker. I also hated going to the gym class because I was often picked last during the team selection, and I had to associate with this other girl.

I was a skinny girl with strawberry blonde hair, cut in a shag, was under-developed, and had acne. My mother made me wear hand-sewn knee-high skirts to school when the fashion was to wear miniskirts and jeans. Some of my pants were so short they could be considered "floods." I felt like an outcast and was very lonely.

In eighth grade, I finally redeemed myself. I wore nicer clothes, was taking medicine for my acne and learned to play well in gym class. Despite these improvements, I remained quiet and associated with a few loyal friends.

When I started high school, I longed to try different extracurricular activities. I wanted to try out for the operetta, but I still didn't have the courage. I tried out for basketball, but unfortunately, the second night I became ill.

I regrettably resolved to bury myself in my school work. I never dated and rarely talked to boys. I was never asked to a dance or attended my junior or senior proms. I hardly went to any of the games in school. Unlike other girls, I only went to one pajama party. As you can see, I led a very sheltered life.

My mom insisted I take a bunch of secretarial courses, which I hated. One of our business teachers would threaten us if we looked at the keyboard of the typewriter. Driver's Education was another class I dreaded. I barely passed the written test. My practical experience was short-lived; I drove with a male gym teacher and several cool boys. I was nervous, in fact, the male teacher never even let me pull out of the parking lot! I end up quitting because my mom didn't want me to jeopardize my skills in Secretarial Office Practice. This was such a letdown. I had to wait another three years for my dad to teach me to drive because he wanted to teach my sister and me simultaneously.

When I was sixteen, I almost attempted suicide. Previously, I had made the following statement, "I will be pretty when I turn 16." That day when I woke up in my bedroom, my mom and my sister came in and started laughing. My mom jokingly said, "Are you pretty today?" That was it, I was done. I ran into the bathroom opened up the closet door and looked for the sleeping pills. I was just about to open the bottle when suddenly, my sister barged in and slapped the bottle from my hands.

In my junior year, my mom encouraged me to take journalism. I really liked my teacher, and she liked my

172

work. In fact, she encouraged me to pursue writing for a career. I took the SATs, but my scores were low. So with no direction and not much confidence, I took the summer of '79 off and then went job hunting.

After working with a few temp agencies in Philadelphia, I landed an office job. This job was definitely not right for me. My mom advised me to quit, and so I did. I was called for a second interview at Woolco, a department store in Turnersville, NJ. They hired me immediately. Retail was a good career for me. This job propelled me to come out of my shell and gain confidence. I started dating at this store and eventually, I was engaged to one of my co-workers. I worked at that store until it's closing - a very sad time for everyone who worked there.

In addition, my relationship with my fiancé wasn't going well. He became possessive, critical, and demanding. The turmoil of my engagement, besides losing my job, made it difficult for me to sustain another job. I became withdrawn and nervous again. I expressed to my fiancé I wanted to see a therapist; he didn't understand the urgency of me seeing a professional. I also was dealing with serious issues regarding my mother.

I often experienced worry, fear, anxiety, nervousness, lack of confidence, excessive crying, seasons of depression and mild panic attacks. Many factors contributed to my emotional rollercoaster throughout

173

the years.

The first factor was my upbringing. My father would joke around or exaggerate excessively. He also worried often. My mother was very paranoid, and I noticed this more after I graduated from high school. She refused to teach me household chores and wouldn't allow me to use the major appliances. She also would lose her patience and start yelling or hitting me. My mom puzzled me, sometimes, I couldn't figure out what I did wrong. My mother also tried to discourage me from pursuing other job positions. For several years, as an adult, I felt like I was walking on eggshells around her.

I did my best to listen and obey my parents. My parents were not very supportive or encouraging, in fact, they just instilled the fact that I was a fragile and shy girl that needed guidance and protection. I didn't start speaking up for myself until my early twenties. I lived in my sister's shadow. She was pretty, intelligent, sociable, talented and strong-willed. She excelled in the band, drama, and academics; my parents really encouraged and supported her.

The second factor was my religious background. My mom and dad didn't bring us up in the Lord. I viewed the Catholic Church as a bunch of rules, traditions, and holidays. We also didn't attend youth events after we received Confirmation. When I married, I converted to a Lutheran like my husband.

The third factor, I already mentioned in great detail, was my academic and social experiences. I had a great deal of negative energy around me, along with several traumatic events that happened. Later in life, I sensed disapproval, negativity, and competition from several coworkers.

The fourth factor was my view of myself and the inner voice that tormented me. I broke up with my fiancé, over the holidays in 1984. I also did some self-help on my own. I took out a book from the library entitled "The Inner Enemy: How to Fight Fair With Yourself." This book helped, but more healing was done several years later when I asked God to help me forgive my mom. I also did an extensive study on forgiveness from reading a recovery bible. On two occasions after we moved back home from North Carolina, as part of my healing journey, I was led to forgive everyone in my entire life who hurt me through their words or actions.

In my late thirties, my mom began to appreciate me more. Oh, there was one scary incident a week before my wedding shower in 1990, where she attacked me in my bedroom closet! I slept in the car and the next day ran away, first to my girlfriend's house and then to my fiancé's house. I got very sick! I wanted to elope. My new fiancé wanted me to have a nice wedding. The breakup with my first fiancée was hard on me. Memories would flood my mind. I eventually let them go.

One of my classmates invited me to a nondenominational meeting. I was hesitant, but I went. At this meeting, there was a kind Minister who talked about the importance of establishing a relationship with God. continued to go to the meetings, fellowship nights and retreats. I dated a few guys. I felt accepted in that fellowship; it was a safe place. I even started reading the Bible.

After about two years later, I wanted to find my true love. I started going to the bars with my girlfriends and dating guys from the classifieds. Unfortunately, I never found Mr. Right. I never found Mr. Right, even after I went on a cruise with my girlfriend to Bermuda. I decided I would let fate take its course. Soon after I made this decision, I saw a classified ad in a shopper's guide. It was an ad for Christian singles meetings Christian singles. To make a long story short, this is where I met my husband. He only lived 15 minutes away in a small town I never heard of. We married on September 22, 1990.

After the closing of Woolco, I went from job to job. Nothing ever lasted. Finally, in 1987, I landed an office job at an employee benefits company in Philadelphia and worked there for six years. The job went very well.

In 1993, I developed Irritable Bowel Syndrome

because the job had become stressful. On top of all my filing work and other duties, I was now responsible for filling in as the receptionist, because our long-time receptionist quit. This was frustrating to me personally and to the president of the company because we could never find an adequate replacement. I decided that I could no longer work there, and I wrote my letter of resignation. My husband had a job in retail, he was a great worker and had steady employment. I was going from job to job. I would either quit, get fired, or the company would close. This left our finances unstable.

In 1996, we left New Jersey and move to North Carolina. My husband found a similar job in retail. I took a job at a Hallmark store. I worked there briefly and then quit. I had challenges working with the manager. Then my vicious job cycle started up again. I worked in retail or office positions.

When I was 39 years old, I had our beautiful baby girl Christina. My husband let me stay home until she enrolled in kindergarten. In 2003, my husband and I attended a business conference. Sunday morning, we both walked down the aisle and willingly surrendered our hearts to Jesus. We didn't have a home church, but we visited a certain non-denominational church when they held special events. Shortly after this business event, we joined a local church. I helped with the children's ministry.

177

I started college in 2007 and pursued a degree in Early Childhood. I worked as a homeschool assistant for a few months but was let go, because the employer had financial difficulties. I worked in a couple of preschool positions. Unfortunately, they never lasted, because of indifferences I had with the teacher or the director of the facilities.

During this time, our church was having a breakthrough course administered by a Christian therapist. The participants had to choose a particular part of their lives they wanted to change. I chose to break my endless job cycle. It was difficult to share my thoughts in a group setting, so I took it by myself. The course helped me; it made me feel worthy again.

In 2009, my family moved back home to New Jersey, and we stayed. My husband's disability was finalized; he was declared visually impaired. I continued my education and received my degree. College was great! I excelled in most of my courses, was accepted in two honor societies, and gained more confidence. Unfortunately, I still couldn't keep a job.

Finally, in the fall of 2015, I was just fed up. I was ready to draw the line in the sand, and I knew I had to become a confident person. In addition, to my already long list of uncontrollable emotions, I also noticed that I had developed performance anxiety, perfectionism and comparison tendencies. Once I made that decision, God began to move. I got grounded in what the Bible says, and through a corporate fast from my church, God associated me with Godly women who were successful and confident.

Through my faith journey, I began to focus more on what God said and didn't put people's opinions above the Scriptures. I also started seeing myself as God sees me. He sees me as a special person. I have learned that I was a highly sensitive person, meaning I had sensory issues and a sensitive spirit.

I had to know my true identity in Christ, but I also had to be content with my personality - and now, I am.

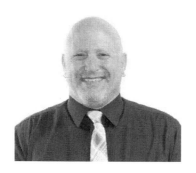

Al Levin

Al Levin is married and has four children. He is an assistant principal in a public elementary school and has been in the field of education for nearly twenty years. He has completed all of the coursework for a Co-Active coaching certificate through the Coaches Training Institute. The coaching work has allowed him to support the staff he works with in the public schools, as well as others who are seeking support in reaching their goals or working past challenging times in their lives.

He is someone who has recovered from a major depressive disorder, an illness that was quite debilitating for nearly six months of his life. Through this experience, he has become very passionate to learn more about mental health and supporting others with a mental illness; particularly men with depression. He speaks publicly for the National Alliance on Mental Illness (NAMI) and on his own. He has a blog that focuses on depression, other forms of mental illness and suicide prevention. He has a podcast in which he interviews men who have dealt with depression and or other diagnoses. His blog and podcast can both be found at TheDepressionFiles.com. You can also find him on Twitter at @allevin18.

He has been published in *The Mighty*, *The Huffington Post*, and *Psych Central* and featured in *Esperanza Magazine*.

A School Administrator's Experience With Major Depression

By Al Levin

"You may know their name, but probably not their story".

"Have kindness...always".

Several years ago, my career took a large leap from an assistant principal in a public elementary school to becoming the principal. This was an exponential increase in the amount of responsibility that was put upon me. Instantly, there were many new challenges that I had to face on my own.

I quickly felt overwhelmed. My stomach had a continual knot in it and I could hardly eat anything at all. I threw away entire meals. My sleep began to suffer. I would roll around in bed, my mind racing, unable to fall asleep until near morning. I would try to sleep with my iPhone on, earbuds in, playing beach sounds. I would do anything at all to fall asleep. I needed sleep so desperately, yet found it nearly impossible to get any at all. I shared my feelings with my brother, a family doctor, who tried his best to support me from overseas, where he was living.

I sat in administrative meetings before the school year even began, wondering how I would accomplish all that needed to be done. I would drive down the highway at a snail's pace, literally going no more than fifty miles an hour, dreading the arrival to the school where I knew that I wouldn't even know where to begin, as it seemed there was so much to accomplish. I started counting down the days that were left in the school year when we were only in October.

I finally decided that I could do this no longer. I made an appointment with my family doctor. This, alone, became another stressor. How could I not be at the school that I was trying to lead? At my doctor's appointment, I could not even sit down. The doctor came in, shook my hand, and took a seat on his leather swivel chair while I paced back and forth in the tiny clinic room.

This was so strange to me. I'm not someone who paces. I couldn't stop myself and the doctor, who had been my doctor for many years, immediately knew something was wrong. I spoke to him of my previous three or four weeks; the stress, lack of sleep, not being able to eat and the overall feeling of not being myself. He gave me a questionnaire and made a

183

quick diagnosis of "Situational Depression." He prescribed medicine and told me I should probably see a psychologist.

Leaving the doctor's office, I felt more stressed than ever. I called my mother from the car to tell her I would have to contact the superintendent and resign from my position. I told her I could no longer take the stress. She urged me to think about it before making any rash decisions. I took her advice.

Even with the start of medication, I was not feeling like myself at work and I was not sleeping any better. I continued to keep my brother in the loop. He emailed me an article from a well-respected medical journal that encouraged doctors who prescribed antidepressants to also prescribe a low dose of a particular benzodiazepine. During the day, the benzodiazepine would help with anxiety and depression. Before bed, a slightly larger dose would help with sleep. This was primarily used as a buffer until the antidepressant started working, as antidepressants often take four to six weeks before they have much effect. I brought the article to my family doctor and shared my brother's thoughts with him. Luckily, he agreed to add the benzodiazepine to my regimen of medicines. Finally, I was getting a better handle on my sleep.

I continued taking the medicine, and I began to see a therapist. I found my first therapist to be more depressing than helpful. I wanted to give therapy a real shot, so I continued for two more sessions. After these sessions and still feeling no connection, I decided I would look into others. I found another therapist, and this one included the bonus of scheduling evening appointments. Scheduling appointments during my work hours would only cause me more stress and add to my depression and anxiety.

I was able to survive my first year of the principalship and my mental health seemed to be gradually improving. During the summer after my first year as a principal, my wife and I had twins. This doubled the number of children in our family. We now had a fiveyear-old, a three-year-old, and two newborns as I entered my second year as a principal. This year, I could have more support through the district; a mentor and a leadership coach who worked with me and our school Leadership Team. This second-year seemed to go much smoother. My direct supervisor was rarely in the school, which led me to believe that the building was running smoothly. However, at my final review, to my surprise, my supervisor informed me he would ask me to do a third year of probation. This was not as bad as being non-renewed, but not as good as being granted tenure. His reason was that he only had one year to work with me and to mentor me. Having rarely seen my four children for two years, leaving home before they were awake and regularly getting home after dinner and often after bedtime, I requested a voluntary demotion.

My first year back as an assistant principal came and went without much excitement. For whatever reason, mid-to-late October 2013, my body began to feel strange. It was a heavy, lethargic feeling as if moving through quicksand all day long. I emailed my brother right away and shared this information with my best friend and my wife. I didn't realize it but this was the start of what would be a very deep, dark depression. One that words cannot fully describe. My brother would later share with me that my first email to him describing these changes was at almost the exact time, three years earlier to when I shared the start of my 2010 depression with him.

Every little thing that went wrong at the time would feel like the world was crashing down on me. I didn't want to leave the house for any reason at all. I was fearful that someone would see me during the day while I was out and might ask or wonder why I wasn't at work. Not only that, but motivating myself to get out of the house was nearly impossible. The few times I made it out of the house, my wife was left wondering if I would make it back home.

When I returned to work, I stayed in my office for much longer periods of time, as this became my safe place at work. If I didn't venture out of the office, perhaps I could minimize my interactions with staff.

186

When I had conversations with staff, I always unintentionally put a negative spin on things and then blamed myself.

After a week and a half of winter break, more struggling with no structure, and seeking isolation and the safety of being in bed behind closed doors much of the time, it was time to go back to work. I somehow managed three more weeks. The days became more challenging at work. I had more isolation and more crying bouts in the evenings. Any new task that came my way, no matter how small it may have been, felt like an additional huge weight upon me, an insurmountable mountain to climb. I tried my best to get out of the office and into classrooms.

I was meeting with my psychologist weekly at this point. I was also on a new medication that my psychiatric physician assistant had prescribed. I hoped that things would get better. However, they did not. I was experiencing more frequent suicidal thoughts. At one of my psychiatry appointments, I specifically asked if these thoughts could be due to the medication, as suicidal thoughts are indicated as a possible side effect of many antidepressants, as ironic as that may be. The physician assistant's response was, "It could be the medication or it could be the depression." He increased the dosage of my medication at that appointment, hoping to have a better outcome. However, my suicidal thoughts

187

became much more frequent throughout the day and much more planned out. One night, I woke up even dreaming of my plan. This scared me to the point of making an emergency psychiatric appointment, temporarily leaving work, and checking myself into a partial hospitalization program for three weeks.

The Recovery

Gradually, with some bad days here and there, and with a lot of effort, I continued to get better and better mentally each day. I was told by one psychologist that it takes a minimum of one year to fully recover from a major depressive episode. I would agree. It took me about two years to feel completely recovered.

I continue to work at maintaining my mental health through various avenues. I continue to go to support groups for both anxiety and men's depression. I have a psychologist who I trust and know that I could schedule an appointment with at any time. I continue on medication and see a psychiatrist twice a year. I try to exercise on a regular basis and maintain a healthy diet. I continue to pull out the pastels now and then to create art with my kids and I have picked up the guitar. I try to be fairly consistent with meditation and mindfulness. I journal on a somewhat regular basis. I have found that supporting others with depression has been very therapeutic for me. I am connected with other men who I support and I have been trained by the National Alliance on Mental Illness (NAMI) as a speaker to share my story and to lead anti-stigma presentations.

Having gone through this major depressive episode has changed me in many positive ways. I have learned a great deal about mental illness, particularly depression. I realize that I had awful stereotypes in my mind regarding people living with mental illnesses and now I understand that it can hit anybody, any race, from any socioeconomic group. I have become very passionate about working towards minimizing (or even eliminating) the stigma around mental health, supporting men with depression, suicide prevention and awareness, and changing what I consider to be a broken mental health system.

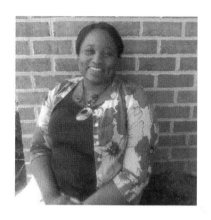

Chou Hallegra

Chou Hallegra is a best-selling Author, a sought-after Speaker, a Certified Life Coach, and a multi-credentialed Mental Health and Ability Consultant. She is passionate about helping people rise above their circumstances and enjoy life to the fullest. When she is not training, writing, counseling, coaching, or speaking, you'll find her exploring new towns, museums, and historical sites with her children. Chou is originally from Brazzaville, Congo and has made South Central Pennsylvania her second home.

Find out more about Chou and her work at www.graceandhopeconsulting.com.

Living On Purpose: From A Psychiatric Unit

To A Fulfilling Life

By Chou Hallegra

"When we turn our stumbling blocks into stepping stones, we find joy in the journey"

– Chou Hallegra

"Hello, my name is Chou. I'm a depression, anxiety and trauma survivor."

This is part of my story that I want to always remember. I currently support others who are experiencing these challenges and although it might be one of the hardest things I have ever done in my life, I love every minute of it.

I will never forget how I entered this field – not as a counselor, a therapist, a trainer, or a consultant - but as a peer. No matter how many degrees, certifications, and accomplishments I might have, I don't want to ever forget that I am a person with mental health challenges myself.

Keeping this front and center helps me meet people where they are, simply because I have been there. Everything I have learned through my years of formal training will never replace what my lived experience has taught me. I have had counselors who knew a lot about mental health and psychology but still didn't get it. I'm honored to both "know it" and "get it." And for that, I will forever be grateful.

I first became aware of my mental health needs at the age of 24. I was a first-time mom living in a new country with not much support. I found myself surviving and not living and I decided that was not the life I wanted. I wanted more out of life. In that moment of desperation, I decided it was time to seek help.

It was important for me to find a provider who not only could help me with my mental health symptoms but also respected and valued my belief and incorporated that into my treatment plan. That turned out to be harder than I thought. I had counselors who respected my values but couldn't help me incorporate them into the services I was receiving. I also had good friends who shared my values but didn't know how to support me on my mental health journey. I was somewhat forced to keep the two separated and that bothered me.

I remember picking up the phone and calling local mental health agencies. A couple of weeks later, I went to my first counseling session and connected well with the therapist. I felt comfortable talking to her and I left every session feeling lighter than I did when I first arrived (at least emotionally). She listened and asked questions that forced me to think about things I didn't consider before. I felt respected, valued, and even validated.

I wondered if talking to another human being could be that therapeutic, how come we as humans don't do much of that? I came to understand that it's not just talking to another human being that's actually therapeutic. The person has to be willing to listen – not just listen to what I'm saying, but also to help me process the things that I didn't know how to put into words. My therapist made me feel like a million-dollar when I actually felt less than a penny – that feeling is something I now want to leave with everyone I meet. Through both my work and my personal life, I intentionally go the extra mile to let people know that they matter and that they are worth my time.

Recently, I canceled business meetings and drove through a couple of counties, just to go share coffee and a muffin with a young man who needed that reminder. It took me two hours to help him finish that snack and every minute of it was worth it. The smiles, the look in his eyes and the hugs, all said, "thank you for being here." This young man doesn't use words to communicate but everything in him was speaking. Moments like this are what I strive to create. And I learned this when I was the client, the patient, the consumer - and not the professional. **If everyone knew that they matter, at least to one person, I guarantee that suicide rates will drastically decrease.**

Back to my experience as the counselee, when I sat at the other end of the table. I continued seeing my therapist weekly and a month or so later, I also started seeing a psychiatrist at the same practice. The psychiatrist started me on some antidepressants and one of them wasn't working so well for me. It can take some time to find the right dosage and it takes at least two to three weeks to feel the effect of the medication in your body.

One afternoon, I found myself in my bedroom overwhelmed by the desire to die. I was done. Life was too hard. I felt like I had tried everything I could. I thought it would be easy to just vanish. I told myself my family didn't care about me and nobody would even notice that I was gone. I kept thinking this will put an end to the pain and I can finally reach my happily ever after.

Looking back, I now realized that it wasn't so much that I wanted to die but rather I no longer had the strength to live - living was just too hard. This is what depression does to us. Every little thing becomes a giant to fight, a mountain to climb, and I had no strength to do either one of those things. At least, if I died, then I wouldn't have to work so hard to just be alive.

These thoughts went on and on in my mind like a record player on continuous play. I didn't know how to stop the tape. Thankfully, I already had a counselor. I had a number to call. So instead of taking the entire bottle of pills that I was holding in my hand, I picked up the phone instead and called my counselor. She advised me to go to the nearest emergency room right away. I trusted her – remember, she is the one who made me feel like a million-dollars, so I followed her advice.

I drove myself to the hospital and went straight to the emergency department. After spending a few hours in the emergency room, talking to a crisis worker and being examined by medical professionals, I was transferred to a psychiatric hospital. **Five days in that facility felt like FOREVER, yet that's what I needed at the time. My mental health recovery started there, in a psychiatric hospital.**

People often think that recovering is being without symptoms, without urges, and that's not true. Recovery is not a linear road. It's made of ups and downs. Sometimes recovery is three steps forward and two steps backward. Some days, it's dancing in the rain, and on other days, it feels like being stuck in the mud. But as long as you stick to it, then you're in recovery. **It's not how many times you fall that**

matters. What counts is how often you rise up.

At the end of my hospital stay, I was released to continue with outpatient therapy and psychiatry. But internally I needed something more, something bigger than myself, something that will keep me going, that will motivate me every single day to get out of bed. I only had one child at the time, my daughter, and thank God I had my daughter because she was the reason why I didn't take those pills the day I felt so suicidal. I did not want her to go grow up without a mother and I chose to live, just for her. **I had nothing left to fight but I told myself that I could try, at least one more time, just for her**.

Life after my hospitalization was hard. Depression and anxiety have a way of sucking the life out of you. I needed something that was worth living for, something beyond just my daughter. Since I made the decision to live, I told myself I better be living and not surviving. I didn't want to go back to the girl who just went through the motions with no emotions. I was tired of numbing my way through life.

I realized that what I needed was to not just find my purpose but to actually live on purpose. I decided to be very intentional about the kind of life I was living. Every single day I had to remind myself that I wanted to live a meaningful life. At first, it felt like I had to make that decision every second. Months of therapies turned into years of support and maintenance, and I slowly started feeling better.

I eventually started feeling happy enough to think about my future. I pursued my undergraduate and graduate education, and went on to become a Board Certified Christian Counselor, a Certified Family

Trauma Professional, and a Certified CognitiveBehavioral Group Therapist, among other things. I now offer the integrated support I was looking for during my lowest moments. If I needed it, I'm sure many more do as well. And the past few years have proven this to be true.People reach out to me for one thing and before we know it, we are working on "all the things" and they appreciate that I can provide effective support that meets more than just one need. Grace & Hope Consulting, LLC might not be called a "one-stop-shop" yet, but it's turning out to be one for many individuals and their families.

My personal experience with mental health challenges has helped me become a voice for people with mental health concerns and a beacon of hope for so many more. My days are not all glory, my life is not perfect, but I live *on* purpose. **Today, I no longer live just for me, I live so that others may live.** I now have the tools I need to stay mentally and emotionally well and I ought to share these tools with others who desperately need them. When life starts to get to me, I pull out a tool out of my wellness toolbox and address the issue, rather than feeling trapped in my circumstances.

I'm sharing all this to remind you that your life is worth living. Even when you feel like you don't have the strength to go on, even for just one more day, just show up. Show up tomorrow and the day after and the day after that. Before you know it, you would have lived longer than you thought possible.

Also, don't suffer alone. If I had never reached out for help, I wouldn't be here and you wouldn't be reading this story. If I have died by suicide back in 2008, I would have missed out on so many things, things that I couldn't even imagine would happen in my life. Now that they happened, I can't imagine my life without them.

In the past eleven years, I had two more kids who are very funny, adventurous and awesome teachers to everyone they meet. I have also had the privilege to build a strong bond with my daughter and watch her become one of the most caring and wise teenagers I have ever met. I also became a best-selling author multiple times, spoken on multiple stages and platforms, and touched so many lives – many of those I would never meet.

Your life is worth living and live it to the fullest. Just take those baby steps and keep finding new ways to stay on your wellness journey, even if it's just one single thing you can do each day. Sometimes, seemingly simple tasks can create a ripple effect that gives your life meaning and purpose, or simply the motivation to live one more day – either way, you win at the end.

The world needs all of us to share our stories. We have shared ours here and I hope you will share yours as well, all around you and across the globe. Let's break the stigma, one story at a time!

RESOURCES

Top HelpLine Resources

- <u>Anxiety and Depression Association of America (ADAA)</u> provides information on prevention, treatment and symptoms of anxiety, depression and related conditions (240-485-1001)
- <u>Children and Adults with Attention-Deficit/ Hyperactivity Disorder (CHADD)</u> provides information and referrals on ADHD, including local support groups (800-233-4050)
- <u>Depression and Bipolar Support Alliance (DBSA)</u> provides information on bipolar disorder and depression, offers in-person and online support groups and forums (800-8263632)
- <u>International OCD Foundation</u> provides information on OCD and treatment referrals (617-973-5801)
- <u>National Center of Excellence for Eating Disorders (NCEED)</u> provides up-to-date, reliable and evidence-based information about eating disorders (800-931-2237)
- <u>Schizophrenia and Related Disorders Alliance of America (SARDAA)</u> offers Schizophrenia Anonymous self-help groups and toll-free teleconferences (240-423-9432)
- <u>Sidran Institute</u> helps people understand, manage and treat trauma and dissociation; maintains a helpline for information and referrals (410-825-8888)

- <u>Treatment and Research Advancements for Borderline Personality Disorder (TARA)</u> offers a referral center for information, support, education and treatment options for BPD (888-482-7227)

Finding Treatment

- <u>Psychology Today</u> offers a national directory of therapists, psychiatrists, therapy groups and treatment facility options
- <u>SAMHSA Treatment Locator</u> provides referrals to low-cost/sliding scale mental health care, substance abuse and dual diagnosis treatment (800-662-4357)

Suicide And Crisis

- <u>The American Foundation for Suicide Prevention</u> provides referrals to support groups and mental health professionals, resources on loss, and suicide prevention information (888-333-2377)
- <u>The National Domestic Violence Hotline</u> provides 24/7 crisis intervention, safety planning and information on domestic violence (800-799-7233)
- <u>The Suicide Prevention Lifeline</u> connects callers to trained crisis counselors (800-273-8255)

Financial Assistance

- <u>Allsup</u> provides non-attorney representation when applying for SSDI (800-279-4357)

- <u>HealthCare.gov</u> provides specific information about coverage options in your state, including private options, high-risk pools and other public programs (800-318-2596)
- <u>Needhelppayingbills.com</u> provides information on state and local assistance programs, charity organizations and resources that provide help paying bills, mortgage assistance, debt relief and more
- <u>NeedyMeds</u> provides information on available patient assistance programs (800-503-6897)
- <u>Partnership for Prescription Assistance</u> helps qualifying individuals without prescription drug coverage get the medications they need

Advocacy And Legal

- <u>Legal Services Corporation</u> provides civil legal aid to low-income Americans. Use their website to find programs in individual states. Scroll to the bottom of their website to find locate legal aid near you
- <u>National Bar Association</u> provides a directory of state and local bar associations to help find legal representation
- <u>National Disability Rights Network</u> protects the civil rights of individuals with disabilities, particularly in hospitals and state prison systems. Click on the map on the right-hand side of their website to locate the agency near you

Community Support Services

- <u>Clubhouse International</u> provides a directory of clubhouses. Clubhouses provide opportunities for

education, employment and social activities. Click
the 'International Directory' tab on their website to
find contact information for local clubhouses

- www.homelessshelterdirectory.org provides a
  national directory of homeless shelters, assistance
  programs, soup kitchens and more
- Job Accommodation Network provides resources
  and guidance on workplace accommodations and
  disability employment issues. Their website
  includes a directory of state vocational rehabilitation
  offices (800-5267234)

Research & Statistics

- National Institute of Mental Health (NIMH) provides
  information on statistics, clinical trials and research.
  NAMI references NIMH statistics for our website
  and publications (866-6156464)

** This resource list was created by nami.org

We are rising above depression, anxiety, addiction,
sexual abuse, and other traumas...

SO CAN YOU!!

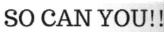

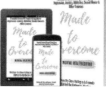

Made in the USA
Middletown, DE
11 April 2023

28462876R10125